CW00925495

REIKI HEALING HANDBOOK

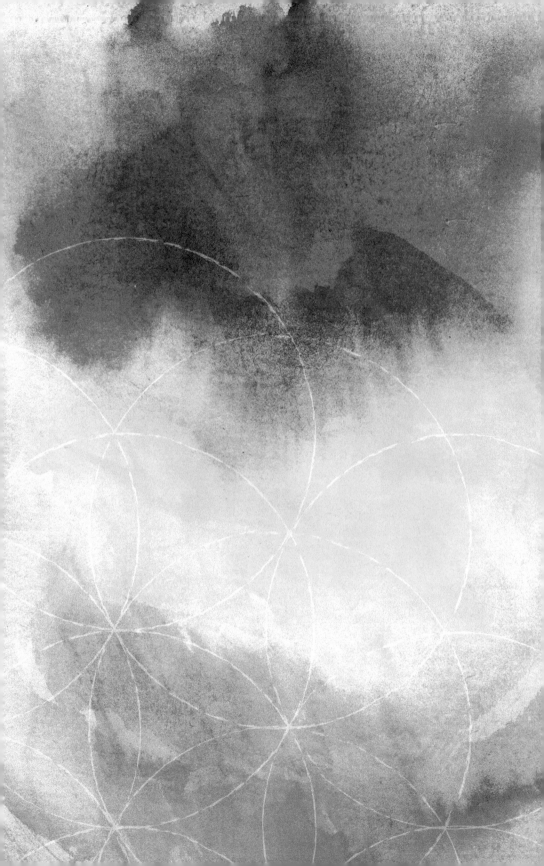

REIKI HEALING HANDBOOK

How to Activate Energy Healing with Chakras, Symbols, and Hand Positions

Nathalie Jaspar and Alena Goldstein

Illustrations by Simona Bortis-Schultz

ROCKRIDGE
PRESS

Copyright © 2020 by Rockridge Press, Emeryville, California

No part of this publication may be reproduced, stored in a retrieval system, or transmitted in any form or by any means, electronic, mechanical, photocopying, recording, scanning, or otherwise, except as permitted under Sections 107 or 108 of the 1976 United States Copyright Act, without the prior written permission of the Publisher. Requests to the Publisher for permission should be addressed to the Permissions Department, Rockridge Press, 6005 Shellmound Street, Suite 175, Emeryville, CA 94608.

Limit of Liability/Disclaimer of Warranty: The Publisher and the author make no representations or warranties with respect to the accuracy or completeness of the contents of this work and specifically disclaim all warranties, including without limitation warranties of fitness for a particular purpose. No warranty may be created or extended by sales or promotional materials. The advice and strategies contained herein may not be suitable for every situation. This work is sold with the understanding that the Publisher is not engaged in rendering medical, legal, or other professional advice or services. If professional assistance is required, the services of a competent professional person should be sought. Neither the Publisher nor the author shall be liable for damages arising herefrom. The fact that an individual, organization, or website is referred to in this work as a citation and/or potential source of further information does not mean that the author or the Publisher endorses the information the individual, organization, or website may provide or recommendations they/it may make. Further, readers should be aware that websites listed in this work may have changed or disappeared between when this work was written and when it is read.

For general information on our other products and services or to obtain technical support, please contact our Customer Care Department within the United States at (866) 744-2665, or outside the United States at (510) 253-0500.

Rockridge Press publishes its books in a variety of electronic and print formats. Some content that appears in print may not be available in electronic books, and vice versa.

TRADEMARKS: Rockridge Press and the Rockridge Press logo are trademarks or registered trademarks of Callisto Media Inc. and/or its affiliates, in the United States and other countries, and may not be used without written permission. All other trademarks are the property of their respective owners. Rockridge Press is not associated with any product or vendor mentioned in this book.

Interior & Cover Designer: Heather Krakora
Art Producer: Karen Williams
Editor: Crystal Nero
Production Editor: Rachel Taenzler
Illustration © 2020 Simona Bortis-Schultz.
Author photo courtesy of © Nina Goffi, YES Studio (Natalie Jaspar).

ISBN: Print 978-1-64611-068-1 | eBook 978-1-64611-069-8

R0

For Janine and Chelo:
Merci and gracias for taking care of me.
—*Nathalie*

For Francine.
—*Alena*

CONTENTS

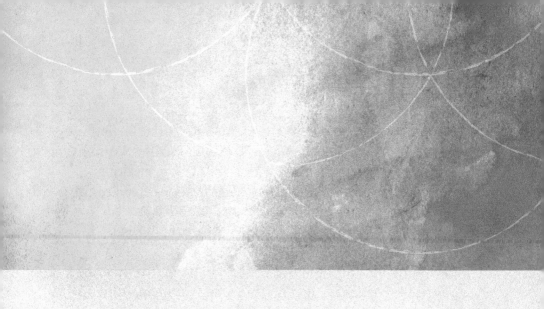

INTRODUCTION

Hello, and welcome! We are Alena and Nathalie, and we are very excited to be part of your Reiki journey. We met at a Reiki class, and from day one we liked each other's energy. Although we approach Reiki practice from totally different places, we share a deep love and respect for this healing system that has allowed our relationship to enrich our practice.

I, Alena, first became interested in alternative healing modalities through yoga. I noticed how it opened me up in ways that had been closed off for years. It transformed my life. Yoga led me to the chakras. Chakras were the first explanation of how my body and the world functioned that made total sense to me. It made me realize that energy, and at least some form of spirituality, is key to our health and well-being. In fact, after working in the field of public health for years, I'd always felt something was missing in our health practices. This prompted me to learn about other healing modalities: acupuncture, sound healing, and, of course, Reiki, in which I trained to the level of Master. I became aware of how inextricably linked this work is to chakra healing. My favorite chakra is Manipura (solar plexus), which is the center of transformation. Through these practices, I have learned to overcome my struggles with confidence, power, and assertiveness—and help heal my digestive disorders.

I, Nathalie, came to Reiki through Google. I am a freelance copywriter, and when work is slow, I like to Google anything that crosses my mind. One day in the mid-2000s, I searched "healing." Reiki came up. At that time, there was little information available, and my first training experiences were less than stellar. Later, I studied with excellent teachers who helped me gain a deeper understanding of this practice and its benefits. I became so in love with Reiki practice that I have sat Level 3 four times and went to Japan to experience some of the original spiritual practices at the root of the Reiki system. You probably have guessed it already—I am a total geek. The frustration of not always finding quality training, and the gratefulness for how Reiki has transformed my life (goodbye drama and migraines), has inspired me to share these precious learnings with as many people as possible.

We joined our experiences to bring you this wonderful handbook. It is not an all-encompassing guide to Reiki knowledge. That is intentional. We wanted this book to be an approachable reference on the basics of Reiki healing and to give you exactly what you need to start a solid practice.

By reading this handbook, you will gain the knowledge of what Reiki is, where it comes from, and, most importantly, how to use it. By no means, however, is it meant to be a substitute for Reiki training. Experiencing Reiki directly with a master and getting attunements are invaluable parts of your journey, and no book can do that.

We are especially excited about a couple of features, specifically how to use Reiki to let go of past traumas and how to use the chakras as guidance for self-healing. Each chakra points to an area that needs support and balance emotionally, mentally, or physically. Combining this guidance with the appropriate Reiki healing tools can lead to a pretty powerful healing experience.

We hope you enjoy reading this book and implementing its ideas as much as we did writing it.

Please note that the recommendations in this book are not intended to cure any disease or replace your current medications. Always consult with your doctor before embarking on a new healing protocol.

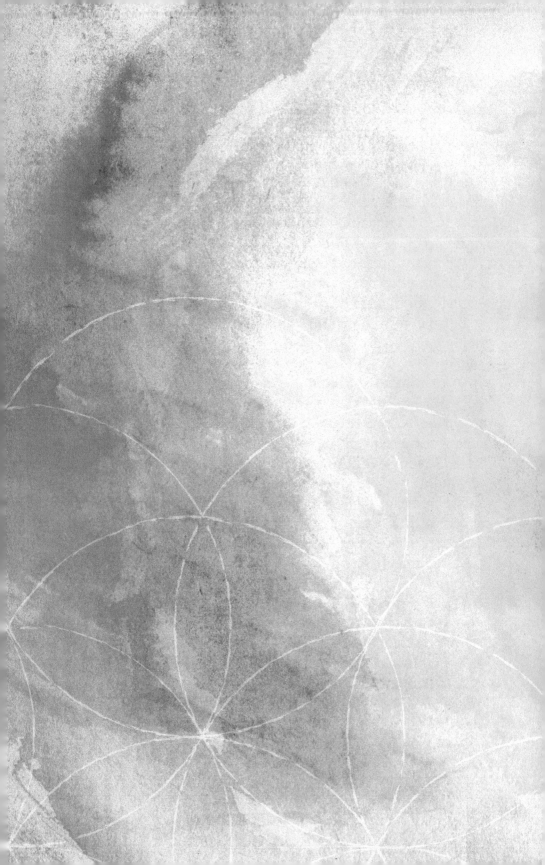

PART ONE

REIKI FUNDAMENTALS

There are no words that can convey the energy, beauty, and depth of Reiki practice. It is something that must be experienced hands-on—literally. However, understanding the elements that make this healing system so unique will give you a strong foundation to build your Reiki practice.

In this section, you will get acquainted with the history of Reiki, the Reiki system of healing, key terminology, levels of practice, the chakras, and the hands-on healing positions.

~~~~~~~

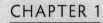

CHAPTER 1

A SHORT HISTORY OF REIKI

The best way to start your Reiki journey is at the beginning: understanding where it comes from. In this chapter, we will give you an overview of Reiki history from when it was developed in Japan to today—when it has become one of the most popular energy healing practices in the world. You will also get an idea of the many Reiki styles available.

But first, let's start with the basics: What is Reiki, what is energy healing, and what are the Five Principles (or Precepts) of Reiki?

WHAT IS REIKI?

Imagine the universe and everything in it: humans, animals, plants, mountains, and even stones. All of it has energy—yes, even the stone! Although invisible, this energy is unlimited and all-encompassing. While science is now demonstrating the impact of energy in our lives, ancient cultures have been aware of this fact for centuries. Known as Chi in China, Ki in Japan, and Prana in India, energy has been and continues to be the basis for many healing modalities.

How does energy healing work? Well, imagine your energy flow is a river. When it flows freely, you function optimally—feeling good, energized, and inspired. However, life's challenges can affect your energy. Worries, fears, anger, and trauma pile up like stones and mud in the river, obstructing its flow until only a trickle is left. You may feel drained and disconnected and can experience physical pain or disease. So, how can you get your energy flowing freely again and, by doing so, jump-start your body's innate ability to heal? Meet Reiki, a century-old Japanese practice that combines hands-on healing and mindfulness techniques to restore the flow of energy, promoting balance and well-being at all levels: body, mind, and spirit.

The word *reiki* can be translated from the Japanese as "universal life force" or "spiritual energy." By connecting more consciously with this energy, or Ki, through the Reiki system of healing, you can feel more relaxed and centered and improve your overall health. You may also start an incredible journey of self-discovery, self-forgiveness, and self-acceptance—letting go of anger and worry to discover a life filled with gratitude and a sense of purpose.

Originally developed as a spiritual practice by its founder, Mikao Usui, Reiki has become one of the most popular energy healing modalities in the West—it's simple, it's effective, and it can be performed by anyone. It is a nonreligious practice. It is also noninvasive, which means it won't interact with medications.

Reiki practice consists of five elements:

1. Precepts—To meditate upon or use as guidelines for the other aspects of the practice.

2. Hands-on Healing—The placement of hands on key points of the body to balance energy.

3. Meditations—To center the mind and build energy.

4. Mantras and Symbols—To connect to more specific types of energies or achieve a determinate state of mind.

5. Attunement—To significantly increase the flow of energy. It is also a way for a Reiki master to transfer wisdom to a student.

All of these—except the attunement, which is performed by a Reiki master—can be practiced on the self. Self-practice is, in fact, the cornerstone of Reiki practice. Because when we heal ourselves, we heal the world. This may sound like a bit much. But think about it: When you feel calm and happy, every person around you benefits from it. You also make more conscious choices at work or as a consumer, thereby helping the whole planet. And it all starts with a simple practice: Reiki.

TRADITIONAL JAPANESE REIKI

The Reiki system of healing was founded by Mikao Usui in Japan in the 1920s. Usui was born to a wealthy Buddhist family on August 15, 1865, and it is believed that he started training at monasteries and martial arts dojos in his youth.

As an adult, Usui was able to travel to Europe, America, and China as a result of the Meiji Restoration, which opened Japan's borders to other nations for the first time in 200 years. He is also said to have achieved the title of a lay monk in Tendai Buddhism (a type of Buddhism that includes esoteric practices) and learned elements from Shinto and Shugendō (Japanese religions with shamanic elements).

In 1922, after years of training in meditation and esoteric practices, Usui went to the sacred Mount Kurama in Japan to sit in a 21-day meditation without food or water. It is assumed that he reached Anshin Ritsumei (enlightenment) during this meditation, and that the capacity for healing came as a consequence.

Once he discovered his newfound ability, Usui set out to create a system that would allow every human being to heal themselves and advance toward enlightenment. In addition to his own techniques, he took many elements that were part of traditional Japanese spiritual practices for centuries and simplified them to make them more approachable. This system would become the base for every Reiki lineage currently in practice around the world.

EARLY YEARS

In April 1922, Usui moved to Tokyo to start a society called Usui Reiki Ryoho Gakkai (The Society for Usui's Method for Healing Using Spiritual Energy). He opened a clinic where he gave classes and provided training. It was here that he developed the system thoroughly. Usui included meditations, scanning, and attunements (Reiju in Japanese) to facilitate the training of practitioners with no previous spiritual background.

In time, Usui developed the Reiki symbols to boost the connection to specific types of energy (heaven and earth) or determined state of mind (oneness and nonduality). He gave many attunements to his students—a practice still popular within the Japanese lineages—to increase their energy and wisdom.

Usui also devised the three levels of teachings, which he called Shoden (the beginnings or Level 1), Okuden (hidden teachings or Level 2), and Shinpiden (mystery teachings or Level 3/Master). He had sublevels in each, which have been subsequently eliminated from most lineages.

With Reiki growing in popularity, he opened a larger clinic in 1925 and started traveling to spread his teachings. He died from a stroke in 1926 during one of these trips. Usui had trained approximately 2,000 students and initiated some 20 masters. Many Reiki practitioners travel to visit his grave and memorial stone at the Saiho-Ji Temple graveyard in Suginami, Tokyo.

After his death, many of Usui's Level 3 students opened their own clinics. Among them was Chujiro Hayashi, a naval officer who was very interested in the health benefits of Reiki. Hayashi started recording which hand positions worked best with each ailment and created a set of guidelines for treatment. At the time, these were meant only for practitioners who could not do energetic scanning. He also made the person receiving the treatment lie down. He developed his own style of teaching, which he then passed on to a Japanese American woman from Hawaii named Hawayo Takata in the late 1930s. Takata brought Reiki practice to the United States, and from there, it spread to the whole world.

Takata, who was initiated as a Reiki master in 1938, opened clinics in Hawaii and traveled to the mainland United States to give classes. Her teachings were vastly simplified because she felt some of the original Japanese methods were too complicated or foreign for the American culture. She eliminated many of the meditations and techniques, focusing almost exclusively on the hands-on healing side of the practice. The goal of the system, based on her direct experience and her training with Hayashi, shifted from a spiritual practice to rediscover one's own true nature (nonduality) toward a focus on physical and mental health, as well as emotional well-being.

Takata trained 22 Reiki masters. These masters, among them her granddaughter Phyllis Furumoto, started traveling around the United States and the world. They taught new generations of practitioners and infused new elements into the practice, like the chakra system, the aura, and crystal grids.

After Takata's death in 1980, the Reiki community grew but also splintered into many diverse schools. Today, it is believed that there are millions of Reiki practitioners and thousands of Reiki masters around the world. Reiki, which had been latent in Japan, had a resurgence. This has prompted an exciting exchange of information between lineages and spurred even more growth.

REIKI TODAY

Currently, it's estimated that there are over 150 different styles of Reiki being practiced all over the world. Although they all trace their lineage to Mikao Usui, many masters have incorporated elements from other natural healing therapies or spiritual traditions.

The truth is, there is no better or worse Reiki and no stronger or weaker Reiki. There are just different approaches and tools to fit the diverse needs of practitioners. For some, a more intuitive approach works best, while for others, a more structured style gives them the right foundation to practice. Here are brief descriptions of seven of the most popular styles of Reiki trending today, organized from the oldest to the most contemporary.

USUI REIKI RYOHO

Usui Reiki Ryoho, meaning "teachings to heal or cure using spiritual energy," is the name Mikao Usui himself gave to his original teachings and school. Today, this lineage refers to the branch that was practiced in secret in Japan from World War II to the 1980s and has been practiced openly since then.

Usui Reiki Ryoho has an emphasis on spiritual development and enlightenment. The approach goes beyond hands-on healing and includes techniques and meditations based on century-old Japanese spiritual traditions. In this school, the energy is not channeled from an external source. The practitioner, like every living being, is part of the universe and, as such, can access an unlimited amount of energy. This lineage doesn't work with chakras or auras. It uses the traditional Japanese energetic centers: earth (*hara*), heaven (forehead), and heart.

Reiki, in this tradition, goes beyond a healing modality: It's a way of life. This style is quickly gaining in popularity and is now being taught in many countries outside Japan.

USUI SHIKI RYOHO

Usui Shiki Ryoho, meaning "system of natural healing," is the traditional Western lineage. It originated from Mikao

Usui and came to the West in the late 1930s via Hawayo Takata. As mentioned in the history of Reiki, Takata simplified Usui's original teachings, taking out many of the meditations and techniques, while placing a strong emphasis on hands-on healing.

When she started training Reiki masters (from the 1960s to her death in 1980), the New Age movement was in vogue. Because of that influence, many of the masters she trained added the elements of chakras and auras to the system. They also included the connection to higher beings, sending healing to the past and the future, and the use of crystals.

Today, this is the most popular and widely found style of Reiki.

KARUNA REIKI

Karuna Reiki was created in 1995 by William Rand, founder of the International Center for Reiki Training (ICRT). Rand defines it as the "Reiki of Compassion" (*karuna* is a Sanskrit word that can be translated to "an action that is taken to diminish the suffering of others"). The practice focuses on awakening universal compassion and a feeling of interconnection with all beings. By facilitating the healing of others, we benefit all beings.

Karuna Reiki is available for any practitioner who has a Level 3 (Master) training. It's given on two levels. The training includes four master symbols and eight treatment symbols. This style also teaches specific meditations to work with the "shadow self," uses tools like toning and chanting, and works with all enlightened beings, physically present in this plane or in spirit.

KUNDALINI REIKI

This style was created in the 1990s by Reiki master Ole Gabrielsen. It combines principles from both the Reiki and Tantric traditions. Its goal is to ignite the Kundalini fire at the base of the spine and create a spiritual awakening in a safe, grounded way. While some Western Reiki schools see spiritual energy as an external source that needs to be channeled into the body, Kundalini Reiki believes this force comes from inside the body.

Kundalini Reiki doesn't use Reiki's traditional symbols or hand positions. The practice is "transmitted" through three attunements, the last one allowing you to pass on the energy to others. The practitioner learns to use earth and heaven energy to promote healing and self-development. As with any other style of Reiki, this branch promotes general healing and stress reduction, yet much of Kundalini Reiki's focus is on karmic/past life healing, birth trauma release, sexual issues, and grounding.

GENDAI REIKI HO

Founded by Hiroshi Doi, Gendai Reiki Ho is a blend of traditional Japanese and Western techniques. Doi himself studied numerous styles of Reiki before training in Usui Reiki Ryoho and coming up with his own vision.

Like many Western-style lineages, this lineage works with chakras, unlike in Japan, where the focus is on one energetic center called *hara* (located three fingers below your belly button). Gendai Reiki Ho treatments follow 12 prescribed hand positions, and the school teaches how to send healing to the past and present, as well as how to develop a connection with higher beings and your higher self.

JIKIDEN REIKI

This style comes from Chiyoko Yamaguchi, a Japanese woman first trained by Chujiro Hayashi in 1938 at the age of 17. She practiced until her death in 2003. In the late 1990s, Yamaguchi decided to pass on her original learnings to the rest of the world. She and her son, Tadao, created a new school and named it Jikiden, a Japanese word that indicates a traditional art passed carefully from master to student without modifications.

Jikiden Reiki doesn't use prescribed hand positions. It teaches practitioners to "scan" the body with the hands to feel where the root of the issue may be. Like the Usui Reiki Ryoho style, Jikiden Reiki goes beyond treatments. The core of the practice is the Five Reiki Principles, or Precepts, which are used to work on the self to be better able to help others.

HOLY FIRE REIKI

This is one of the most recent styles. Introduced in 2014 by the ICRT and William Rand (who also created the Karuna Reiki style mentioned on page 10), it focuses on developing a sense of being deeply loved, healing relationships with others, and replacing worry and fear with feelings of kindness, confidence, vitality, optimism, joy, and peace.

According to Rand, he was guided to create this specific type of Reiki during sessions with his spiritual adviser. The style is based on the idea that the Holy Spirit created a particular type of high-vibration healing energy called Holy Fire, which Jesus first brought to Earth. This practice doesn't consider itself religious, although it uses some terms like *God, Jesus,* and *Holy Fire.* They use these terms from a spiritual point of view.

THE FIVE PRINCIPLES OF REIKI

The Five Reiki Principles, or Precepts, are a series of guidelines for both Reiki and life. They are the foundation of the practice and were the first teaching Mikao Usui shared with his students. Originally written in Japanese, there are many possible translations. This is one of the most common interpretations:

Just for today:

- Do not anger
- Do not worry
- Be grateful
- Practice diligently
- Show compassion to yourself and others

The Precepts are not meant to forbid you from ever feeling anger or worry, rather they are a reminder to listen to these emotions, and then to let them go. They also guide you during your practice, especially when performing hands-on healing: You didn't feel anything during treatment? Do not anger. You are not sure where to place your hands while sharing Reiki with others? Do not worry. Be grateful for the chance to share this precious connection with another being.

How to work with the Precepts:

- Start your day contemplating the Precepts.
- Recite them before hands-on healing to get into the right frame of mind.
- Meditate with the Precepts: Choose one line and repeat it silently in your head. Check your body's reaction. Is there an area where there is pressure, tingling, or a color? Focus on that area, breathe, and observe any changes or insights that pop up.

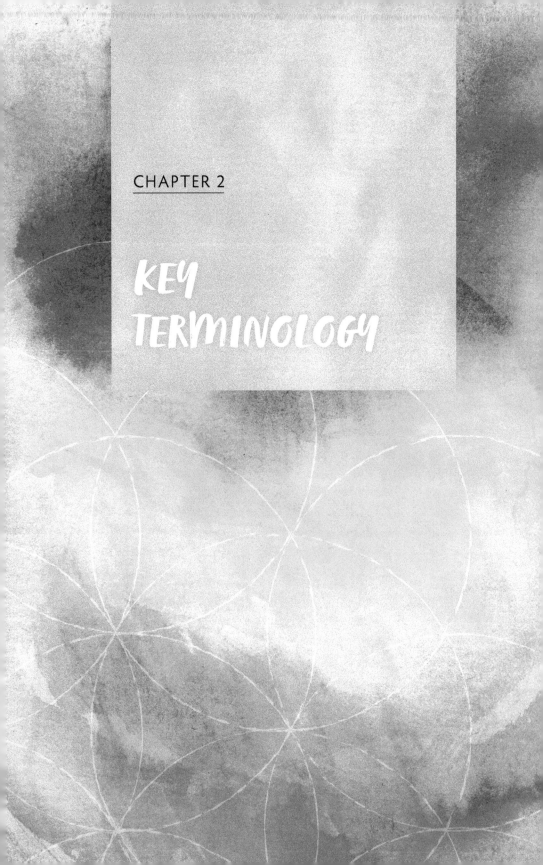

CHAPTER 2

KEY TERMINOLOGY

Before getting into the levels of Reiki training and the different healing techniques, it is beneficial to provide you with a list of terms commonly used by practitioners. Some of these terms, like *hara* and *Gassho*, are native to the original Japanese practice. Others, like *aura* and *chakras*, were incorporated at the time of the New Age influence in the 1970s, and yet others come from more recent healing modalities, such as Donna Eden's Energy Medicine system or moving meditation systems like 5rhythms.

THE LANGUAGE OF REIKI

This key terminology will not only facilitate the use of this book but will also help you navigate the ever-expanding conversation about energy healing in social media and blogs.

Additionally, becoming familiar with these terms and their meanings will help you put into words those fantastic spiritual experiences that are felt with your whole soul but are hard to define.

Please note that many of these words can have multiple definitions and layers of meaning according to their context or the specific healing modality practiced. The aim here is to give the most straightforward explanation and the one closest to the Reiki system. When a particular term has a different interpretation according to the various Reiki styles, it is as close as possible to the original practice in the times of Mikao Usui.

ATTUNEMENT. Also known as Reiju in the Japanese lineages, the attunement is the process in which the master initiates you as a student, sparking a more conscious connection with the universal life force or specific types of energy linked to the symbols. The attunement also gives you the fuel needed to jump-start your energetic practice.

It's almost like you have an inner spiritual battery. The master—through the attunement—charges it so you can start running. Then your daily practice keeps replenishing it. Each successive attunement increases the capacity and sensitivity of your battery, so you can travel further and further in your Reiki journey.

Once you have been attuned, it's for life. You can benefit from further attunements, but they are optional.

AURA. An energy field emanating from the physical bodies of all beings. This energy can be seen by some people as different colors or levels of brightness or clarity, and may offer practitioners insights to an individual's health, mental, and emotional status.

BASIC GRIDS. Basic grids or Reiki crystal grids are an arrangement of crystals (quartz, amethyst, citrine, and others) set with a specific healing intention. Each crystal represents a certain chakra or quality of embodiment (peace, harmony, strength . . . the list of crystals and their qualities is endless). Then, the grid is infused with energy to magnify the healing power. The idea is to keep the energy constantly running through the grid. It is important that the crystals are carefully chosen, properly cleansed, and charged before being used in the grid. The use of crystals in Reiki is not at all necessary for efficacy; however, they are available as a tool for that extra oomph.

BEAMING. Beaming is a form of distance Reiki healing. But rather than being in a totally different place, the person is within close proximity to you (such as across the room or sitting next to you). The Reiki is "beamed" from the practitioner to the individual. Why use beaming? It is believed to work on the auric level and then enters the physical body. It can also increase the energy flow to the client.

BIJA (SEED SOUND). *Bija* means "seed" in Sanskrit and is interpreted to be the origin of everything and the universe. It's the one-syllable sound, or mantra, used in meditation. Each of the different bijas produces a vibration associated with a different chakra. They are used to cleanse the chakras and promote balance. You can either chant the bijas out loud or listen to spoken videos or playlists.

CELTIC WEAVE. Celtic Weave is an energy healing method that was developed by Donna Eden. The palm of the hand traces in a figure eight or infinity shape over the client (a couple of inches to a foot away). Celtic Weave can be used as a technique to promote overall harmony, balance, and unity to one's energy field, similar to the way energy naturally weaves its way through the body. The Ida and the Pingala (major nadis, or energy channels, in the yogic tradition) are actually arranged in this same way, weaving their way through each chakra, from the first chakra to the seventh on opposite sides. Celtic Weave can be applied all over the body or to specific body parts or chakras for attention. Reiki practitioners can borrow this technique and apply it during treatments.

CHAKRAS. Part of the subtle body, chakras are energetic wheels or centers that run along the base of the spine to the crown of the head. Chakras store spiritual and energetic information from the time we are born to the present. Each chakra, depending on its location and qualities, governs our patterns, habits, and how we feel. There are seven major chakras in the Western system, which will be discussed at length below.

GASSHO. *Gassho* means to bring the hands together in prayer as a symbol of union. In the Reiki system, it also means bringing together everything you are with acceptance, and the union of opposites: the masculine and the feminine, the light and the dark, the spirit and the body. Gassho is used to center the mind before treatments, to set intentions, to express gratitude, and to meditate. See the sidebar for how to use Gassho in your daily Reiki practice (page 23).

HARA. While the word *hara* translates to "belly" in English, in Reiki practice it refers to the energetic and spiritual center in the body where one's true essence is found—from where all your energy is sourced. The goal, particularly during meditation, is to connect with the hara to take us back to our true nature and sincere self. The hara is located approximately two inches (or two fingers) below the navel—but focus more on the feeling rather than the exact physical location during your visualizations, moving the energy from the hara to the rest of the body. Symbolically, the hara is also the middle point between the feet and the head—the point at which everything comes together.

You may hear the hara referred to as *Tandien* or *Tanden* (also defined below), which is a Japanese term for essentially the same thing—the place in the body from where life arises.

HEALING. Healing is deeply personal and, therefore, difficult to define in general. Healing can occur on different levels—individual, relational, communal, and universal levels are only some examples. However, within the context of this handbook, healing is defined as the restoration of physical, mental, and/or emotional health—feeling generally vibrant, joyful, and alive. The restabilization and optimization of the flow of energy in the body. As becoming whole.

KI OR CHI. *Ki* (Japanese) or *Chi* (Chinese) translates simply to "energy" or "life force." The Japanese word *ki* is what makes the second part or kanji of the word *Reiki*, and why this word will be used over *chi* for the purpose of this handbook. Everything in the entire world has this ki! Ki is the primary force utilized in Reiki healing and essentially what the practitioner is targeting during a session. Ki is offered from the practitioner to the person receiving treatment.

KUNDALINI. *Kundalini* translates to "coiled snake" in Sanskrit, and it's an energy that sits within each of us at the base of our spine. It rises gradually from the Muladhara (root) chakra all the way up to the Sahasrara (crown) chakra as one reaches spiritual enlightenment. Maybe you've heard of *Kundalini awakening*, which is when this energy rises very rapidly, and it may produce a whole lot of new and intense sensations including but not limited to emotional reactions (releasing blockages, excitement), physical symptoms (changes to sleep, energy, etc.), and increased connection to spirit.

LINEAGE. A Reiki lineage is almost like a family tree. It retraces your line of teachers all the way back to Mikao Usui. A lineage is proof that your Reiki master is formally trained in the Reiki system. It also gives you a clue of your teacher's style (for example, seeing Hawayo Takata in a lineage would most probably indicate Western-style Reiki). Some Reiki masters pride themselves on being closer (in the number of teachers) to Mikao Usui and, therefore, offer a "stronger" Reiki, but that's not necessarily true. Reiki is a practice—hours of work in real life trump being closer to Mikao Usui on paper!

If you study with teachers from more than one lineage, choose the style that represents the way you practice daily. If you decide to blend styles, list the lineages from which you are drawing your techniques.

MANTRAS. A mantra is a word or sound that can be repeated to aid concentration in meditation. In Reiki practice, each type of energy is linked to a symbol and a mantra. The latter is usually used as the symbol's name. In most lineages, the mantras are repeated three times in order to activate the symbols during sessions or meditations. However, the mantras can also be used by themselves for powerful chanting meditations (see the "how-to" in chapter 6 on page 70).

MERIDIANS. Meridians, or *jing-luo* in Chinese, are energy and communication channels that run throughout the entire body and connect to our organs and tissues (and chakras). Traditional Chinese Medicine and acupuncture are based on a system of meridians, through which ki and other materials are flowing. Meridians are also akin to *nadis*, the channels through which prana flows through the body in yoga. These systems are vast and complex and beyond the scope of this book—although the main takeaway is that ki or prana should be flowing freely through the meridians. If the meridians (passageways) are blocked or overloaded, then so is energy, which can translate to a number of different types of ailments.

Note that the meridians deal specifically with energy, not blood flow, which is what makes them a bit more abstract. You can think of them in the same way as you would our bloodstream. Reiki healing can help balance energy flowing through the meridians.

PRANA. Prana is akin to ki but from the yogic tradition. It is a Sanskrit word that translates to "life force." All beings carry prana, and there are five different types of prana or *vayus* (meaning "winds"), which are ways prana can move. Prana vayu is energy moving forward and out, like through our lungs. Apana vayu involves energy moving down and out, like through eliminatory systems. Udana vayu is energy rising and is associated with growth and speech. Samana vayu is heat energy, also associated with things like digestion and absorption, and Vyana vayu is energy circulating throughout the entire body. As you can imagine, the key to good health is having these vayus all flowing optimally.

RADIANT CIRCUITS. Radiant Circuits are meditations, movements, or sequences designed to help restore the flow of energy in the body and promote feelings of joy and positivity.

SCANNING. Also known as Byosen, scanning is defined as the use of hands to "feel" the source of an energetic imbalance or an issue to be worked on during a session. Scanning is done by placing your hands three to four inches above the body and moving them slowly from crown to feet. During this pass, one may feel tingling, warmth, or pulling while hovering over some parts of the body. These signals indicate areas that need treatment. Scanning can be done with both hands or just with the nondominant hand (believed to be more energy-sensitive).

SYMBOLS. The Reiki symbols are visual tools used to connect more consciously with specific types of energy (power/earth, heaven/harmony, distance/heart, and enlightenment). Symbols can be used to reach the right state of mind/energy flow during treatment or a remote session. They can also be used for meditation purposes (grounding, expanding vision, etc.). Like with daily hands-on treatment, the more one uses and meditates with the symbols, the greater one's understanding of the Reiki system. The number of symbols used in practice may vary according to the Reiki style.

TANDEN OR TANDIEN. The *tanden* is the energetic center in the body located inside the hara. It is thought of as the seat of all our energy. It is accessed through deep meditation and focus and can carry energy to the rest of the body. It is okay to use this term interchangeably with the hara.

There are also two other tandens used in Reiki practice—one in the heart space or upper body, and one in the forehead.

A CLOSER LOOK AT GASSHO

Gassho helps center our minds, set our intentions, and express our gratitude before and after treatments. However, Gassho can also be used for meditation, promoting integration, and wholeness. The more whole we feel, the more we heal.

How to meditate with Gassho:

1. Slightly press your palms together in front of your heart, fingers straight.

2. Keep the elbows a little bit away from the body with forearms not quite parallel to the ground.

3. Keep one fist distance between your fingertips and the tip of your nose.

4. Keep your eyes slightly open, focusing on the tips of your middle fingers.

5. Notice your breath, your hands, your body, and any feelings that pop up. You can also visualize white light coming inside your hands and heart in the inhale, and then out as you exhale.

Note: If meditation is new to you, it is okay to close your eyes.

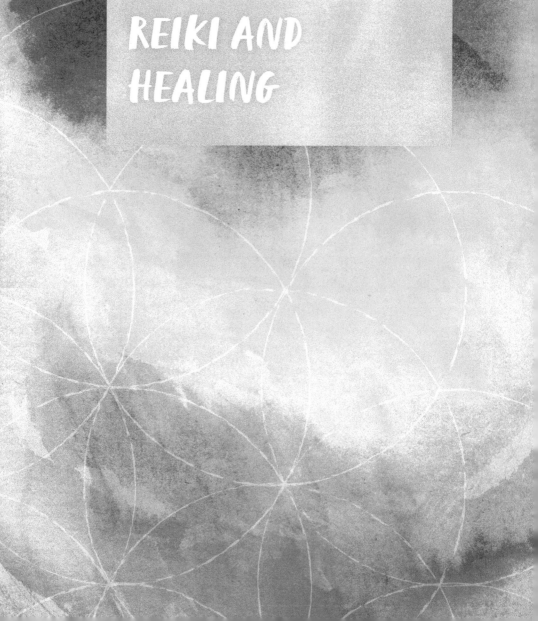

CHAPTER 3

REIKI AND HEALING

Before talking about how Reiki practice works to promote healing, it is important to define healing. Healing doesn't mean just getting rid of symptoms (although that is great!). It means becoming whole, integrating every part of ourselves, and letting go of what no longer serves us. During this process, you may release old traumas, behavioral patterns, and belief systems that are not yours and reconnect with your true essence. Some people define this as "aligning with your higher self." Through the mind-body connection, these benefits translate into the physical world as a healthier and more energized body.

REIKI HEALING BASICS

With the idea of healing through Reiki, it is interesting to note how the Five Reiki Principles or Precepts show you the way: Let go of anger and worry so you can be more grateful. As you practice this with diligence day in and day out, you will feel more compassionate (and connected) to yourself and toward others.

Very nice, but how does Reiki work, specifically? It is a tough question to answer, but the simplest way to explain it is that energy follows the mind. That means wherever you place your awareness—your computer, your cell phone, world problems, a fight with your neighbor—that's where your energy goes. And the more time you spend being aware of things outside your body, or in the past and future, the less energy you have in your body and the present moment. This translates into feeling drained and easily overwhelmed in the best case scenarios, and physically ill in the worst-case scenarios.

Through Reiki, you learn to focus your awareness inward: toward your body, your mind, and your emotions. Hence, your energy is back with you—integrated, flowing, and moving—versus being scattered. The more you practice hands-on healing or Reiki meditations like Gassho, the more aligned your energy is with your mind and your body. You feel more grounded, centered, and energized. This, in turn, helps your body relax and thrive.

Using your hands for Reiki treatments allows you to place your awareness on a particular part of your body, therefore "sending" the energy to that area or chakra. The flow of energy relaxes, softens, relieves, and helps you release what is not needed. If any memory, emotion, or trauma is stored in that area, the Reiki treatment will bring it out to be healed (if you are ready).

Working with chakras can point the way to emotions, areas, or thought patterns that require your awareness and energy to become more balanced. That doesn't mean Reiki won't work if you placed your hand in the "wrong place" or chakra. The energy (and the higher self) has its own intelligence, making the energy flow where it's needed—as long as you remain present.

This is an important thing to keep in mind when performing treatments on yourself, but it's especially useful when facilitating healing for others. Presence, awareness, and compassion while offering a treatment trumps hand placement every time. You just need to be there, focused and open, letting the energy flow, and holding the space for the client to do their own healing. The person receiving the treatment will get whatever they need, and the practitioner will get a crucial life lesson: the importance of letting go of control and entering a state of surrender.

THE BENEFITS OF REIKI THERAPY

The beauty of Reiki is that it activates your body's innate self-healing ability and promotes balance at all levels—physical, emotional, mental, and energetic. During each hands-on healing session, your body and your energetic system will determine what they need to balance, recharge, or release so you can find improved ease and well-being. However, the most commonly reported benefits include:

Reduces stress and anxiety. Reiki is a great way to relax deeply because it soothes your mind and allows your nervous system to shift from "fight or flight" to "rest and digest" mode.

More zzzzz's and better digestion. When your nervous and energetic systems are balanced, you sleep better and wake up more rested, and your digestive system can process food with more gusto.

Helps relieve pain. The warm and soothing qualities of Reiki practice can help muscles relax, relieving pain and discomfort.

Alleviates side effects from medication. This benefit has made Reiki an increasingly popular alternative therapy in cancer hospitals around the United States.

Boosts your immune system. By reducing stress and therefore cortisol and adrenaline levels, Reiki gives your immune system a break so it can function properly.

Promotes detoxing. When your muscles are relaxed, it's easier for the lymphatic system to move the junk out of your body.

Increases energy. By replenishing and balancing your systems and soothing the mind, Reiki allows you to access more energy.

Gives you a renewed sense of hope and purpose. By relieving feelings of overwhelm, Reiki is a great way to reconnect with your sense of purpose and the spark that makes you excited about life.

Better decision-making. Reiki practice makes you more grounded in who you truly are, allowing you to take things less personally, see things more clearly, and make better decisions.

Less reactivity. When you are fully energized, centered, and grounded, it's a lot easier to take a pause before (over)reacting. A pause allows you to breathe and consider: Is it really worth it? Am I making a big ado about nothing? Can I solve this calmly? This leads to. . . .

Less drama. Get ready to say goodbye to toxic relationships and unnecessary complications and to experience more fulfilling personal relationships. Reiki practice makes you feel more centered and boosts self-esteem. This makes it easier to establish healthy boundaries and say no to what's not working in your life.

Hello, intuitive powers. You know that little voice that sometimes sends you messages out of the blue? Messages you know are true, although you have no clue how you know? It's your intuition. Reiki practice strengthens your connection with your inner voice until it becomes loud and clear.

Fills you with confidence. As a consequence of all of the above!

DID YOU KNOW?

An interesting fact about Reiki is that it can be used to heal the past. Many of your memories and emotions are stored in your body, not your brain. During Reiki treatments, you use your hands to reconnect with your energy but also your body (and, hence, memories or feelings). The warm, supportive flow of Reiki helps you process and release them. The more you work on yourself, the freer and lighter your energy will feel.

Two ways to work with the past:
- Before doing a treatment, perform Gassho and set the intent to receive the healing needed—and if that means an issue from the past needs to come up, let it happen.

- Before doing a treatment, perform Gassho and bring a past issue to mind. Feel your body. Is there an area that feels tight, itchy, or different? Place your hands there and let the energy flow.

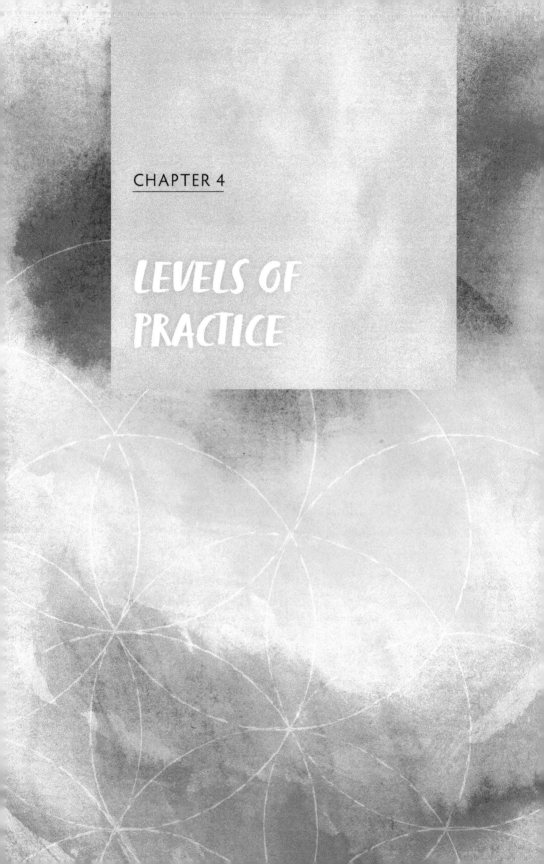

CHAPTER 4

LEVELS OF PRACTICE

When he created the Reiki system for healing, Mikao Usui divided the training into three levels to guide individuals slowly from beginner to mastery. Although he instructed approximately 2,000 students, he initiated very few masters, and advancement was a slow process. Students would practice the tools given at one level for a long time before advancing to the next. Today, Reiki certifications are ubiquitous and offered widely so you can course through the levels as fast as you want. Remember, though: Certifications are great, but practice is the key. Someone who is trained only in the first level, but practices every day, will go further than someone who has completed all levels of certification but practices only once in a blue moon.

~~~~~~~~~~

WHY LEVELS?

Reiki training is commonly divided into Reiki 1, Reiki 2, and Reiki 3, also known as Reiki Master. These levels are intended to give you time to adjust to increased energy flow. Imagine your energetic system like an electric grid: If you infuse it with 10 times the power at once, it will collapse.

Levels also allow you to get the right tools in the proper order to build a solid Reiki practice from the ground up:

- First, do hands-on healing on yourself and your loved ones.

- Second, offer Reiki as a practitioner.

- Last, but not least, perform attunements and teach the Reiki system of healing.

During the training for each level, you will receive a determined number of attunements. As explained in chapter 2 (see page 16), the attunement is a ritual performed by a master on the student to increase energy flow and strengthen the connection to certain types of energies or states of mind associated with four symbols and mantras.

The attunement also points the student toward the next step in her or his Reiki journey.

In spiritual terms, however, the attunement's ultimate goal is to remind you that you and the universe are one.

WORKING WITH A MASTER

Our body's ability to self-heal is innate. Reiki is a system that harnesses this power and intensifies it. Every human can do hands-on healing intuitively, but to learn the Reiki system specifically and understand its depth, you need to start with a Reiki master.

The best way for us to illustrate the value of a Reiki master is to compare it to a GPS. Imagine being left by yourself in an unknown city, let's say Moscow, and asked to go to the main square . . . without a map. You will get there, but it will take you some time, and you may get a little (very) lost along the way. You may even get so frustrated with false turns that you abandon your quest.

A Reiki master provides you with the attunements for Levels 1, 2, and 3 that give you the fuel to jump-start your practice with a taste of what Reiki feels like. By imprinting this feeling in your system, it's easier to find your way on your own. A good Reiki master will also provide guidance when questions pop up during class or later, during your practice.

Reiki masters come in all shapes and lineages. Check the sidebar "Questions to Ask a Reiki Master" (see page 37) for cues on how to find a good match.

REIKI LEVEL 1

Reiki 1 is the first step of your healing journey. At this level, you learn what Reiki is all about, its history, its components, and the basics of how to perform hands-on healing on yourself and others. Depending on the Reiki school giving the training, you will receive either one single attunement or four. You may also learn a few meditations and techniques to promote grounding and energy flow.

This level is all about self-care, reconnecting with your body and your energy, developing sensitivity to its ebb and flow, and slowly releasing layers of anger and worry. Hands-on healing in Level 1 is taught using touch (versus hovering an inch or two above your body) and, in the beginning at least, following prescribed hand positions. These positions cover all the key energetic points in your system so you can focus on developing awareness, and not worry about whether you are placing your hands the right or wrong way (one more example of the Precepts in action).

Although you are taught how to share hands-on healing with others, the focus in Level 1 should be on family, friends, pets, or plants (yes, plants actually love it). It is not recommended to offer treatments professionally at this stage (many insurances won't even cover you yet). In Level 1, you are basically building the foundation of your Reiki house, and you want it to be as solid as possible before putting it on the market.

The length of the training for Reiki 1 varies according to lineages and teachers. Some classes teach it in one day, others in two or three days. If you take a one-day training, check with your teacher to see if it's okay to reach out with any questions that may pop up in your practice (believe us, it will happen).

REIKI LEVEL 2

In Level 2, you learn three symbols and mantras to strengthen the connection with more specific types of energy:

- Earth energy: grounding and focused; related to your connection to life.

- Heaven energy: lighter; related to the spirit, vision, and psychic abilities.

- Heart: compassionate; related to oneness, your interconnection with every living being.

You will receive one or multiple attunements according to your Reiki lineage, and practice how to perform hands-on healing treatments hovering over the body versus touching. You will also learn the protocol to offer distance Reiki sessions to any person or being on the planet. (This is explained further in chapter 7, see page 103.)

Many teachers recommend studying Reiki 2 at least three months after Reiki 1, so you create a strong foundation on which to grow your practice. (Level 1 is required to take Level 2.) As with Reiki 1 training, Reiki 2 is available in one-day classes or multiple-day classes. You can also find a combination of Reiki 1 and 2 training in two days, usually a weekend. Some teachers, however, offer more extended training, requesting that you complete a predetermined number of sessions to complete your certification. Ask yourself what feels best for you. Are you the kind of person who likes to go more in-depth into the tools given, and then slowly grow your arsenal? Or do you prefer to learn more tools and go for the combo class? We are all different. In the end, Reiki is a practice, and what counts is precisely that—how much you practice every day. When you complete your Level 2 certification, you are on the road to offering sessions to others professionally.

REIKI LEVEL 3

Reiki Level 3 is also known as Reiki Master or teacher level. Many teachers recommend waiting six to 12 months after completing Reiki 2 to start the Master level training. You will learn the fourth symbol and mantra from the original Reiki tradition. This symbol and mantra allow the Reiki practitioner to create the energetic space required to perform attunements. The concept of "energetic space" is key. Many Reiki schools have different rituals for attunement, but the space of oneness and the intention behind them are the same:

to remind the student of their connection to the universal life force. You will also learn the specific rituals to perform attunements for the three different levels of training.

You will need completed certifications for Level 1 and 2 to participate in a Reiki 3 training. This level is commonly taught in two- or three-day classes, but many centers offer more extended training to better support students on their road to teaching. Some Reiki masters even offer apprenticeships, where Reiki 3 students act as assistant teachers, gaining valuable direct experience.

Occasionally, Reiki teachers separate this level into two: Advanced Reiki Training, or ART, in which you receive the commonly called Master symbol attunement, and Reiki Master/Teacher, in which you are trained in attuning new practitioners.

Remember: Reiki 3 goes beyond teaching. Although the certification states that you are a master, it's more the representation of a lifelong commitment to the "mastery of the self." In the Japanese tradition, the fourth symbol and mantra stand for "big bright light," or enlightenment. The idea is to reach this state by deepening our understanding through constant practice on yourself and others.

Once you've reached the Master level, you may want to consider re-sitting this class every now and then, taking courses from another lineage, or attending Reiki retreats and "Reiki shares," events where Reiki is offered and received among a community of practitioners. These are great ways to advance your practice and connect with amazing people who share the same passion.

QUESTIONS TO ASK A REIKI MASTER

To receive the attunements and training that will start your Reiki journey, you need a Reiki master. But with so many teachers out there, how do you know if you found the right match for you? Here are a few questions you can ask them to figure it out:

- What lineage do you practice?

- How long have you been practicing? How many years have you been teaching? (Hint: the more, the better.)

- What benefits have you felt in your life from practicing Reiki?

- What is your approach to teaching?

- What will I learn? Will I get a manual and a certificate?

- When I finish the course, will I be able to_____?

- What's your point of view on advancement (going from one level to the other)?

- Do you offer any kind of ongoing support (Reiki shares, one-on-one mentorship, etc.)?

- Can you provide me with testimonials from other students?

Listen to the answers with your head AND your heart. Do you feel at ease? Does the teacher's energy feel loving and supportive? If the answer is yes, then it's a match.

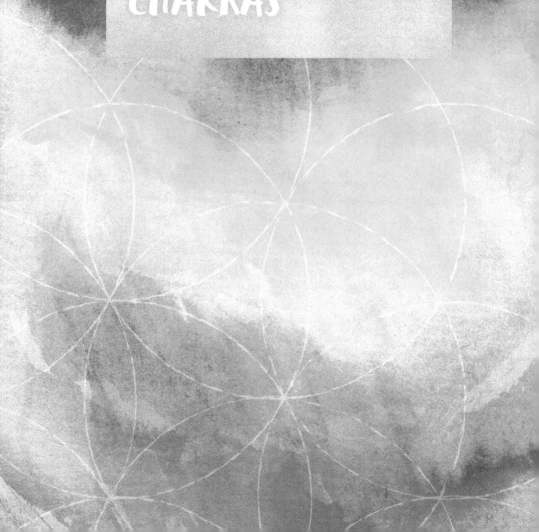

CHAPTER 5

THE SEVEN CHAKRAS

As you can tell by this point, there are many, many approaches to working with energy, and we encourage you to do some more research on the methods and modalities that resonate with your Reiki practice the most. This book focuses on the chakras as the guiding energetic field. Similar to the hara in Reiki, chakras are energetic centers, a part of the subtle body. They store memories and information and, in turn, impact the body and mind. Ideally, energy is flowing freely in and out of the chakras and they are in constant motion. Yet, life experiences, traumas, and transitions of all kinds can cause some disruptions to this motion. Sometimes our minds, bodies, and spirits are affected by these stressors, causing us to become out of balance. Quite commonly, Reiki practitioners will receive requests from recipients to "unblock their chakras," and this can be one of two scenarios—either too much energy is flowing into the chakra (an "excess") or not enough energy is flowing into the chakra (a "deficiency"). Reiki is a great approach to bring back balance. Energy will ultimately flow to where it is needed. However, the chakras and their current state can also be assessed through physical, mental, and/or emotional ailments expressed by clients, and through reading clients auras.

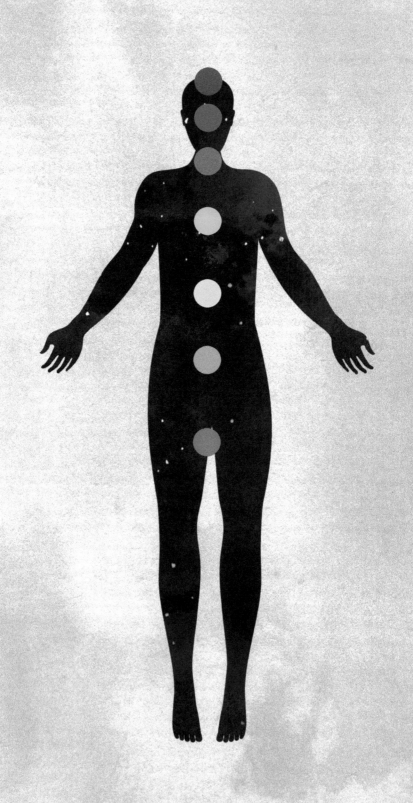

AN INTRODUCTION TO CHAKRAS

Now, let's dive a little bit deeper into the way energy works in the chakra system. In humans, energy flows from the base of your spine to the crown of your head. Spiraling out of the spinal column are the seven major energetic centers (chakras). It should be recognized that some schools of thought maintain only a five-chakra (or five-element) system, while others work based on structures of eight, ten, or more chakras (even 32!). The most utilized and accepted system in the West, particularly for Reiki healing, is seven.

So, where did the chakras come from? And how did they gain recognition in the Western world? Let's start from way back. The word *chakra* comes from the Sanskrit language and translates to "wheel" or "disk." Some chakra experts and healers also refer to them as "wheels of life" or "wheels of light." This traces back to the root word, *cakra*, which stems from the Sanskrit word *cakravartin*, which means "world conqueror or universal king." The cakras actually refer to the wheels of the chariots these conquerors rode. Just as the cakravartins ruled over the world, the chakras are believed to rule over and govern our world—the way we think, feel, and behave. They also correspond to major nerves, organs, and glands, depending where they sit along the spinal column, so their (energetic) health is key to our vitality. Lastly, one more symbolic representation of the chakras you will commonly see in figures or drawings is a lotus flower, with the number of petals corresponding to the specific chakra and having a special meaning. Out of the mud buds a beautiful lotus, but this lotus can be open or closed or somewhere in between.

The chakras are truly linked to yoga practice (or the practice of "becoming one") and were first referenced in the Upanishads (Hindu literature). Here, each chakra is introduced by its original Sanskrit name. The text gives instructions on how one can use the bijas (seed sounds), elements, and deities associated with each chakra at specific positions (points on the body) to meditate and reach nirvana (enlightenment and/or liberation). Many translations of this text have arisen over the years. One of the first in the West was a translation by Arthur Avalon in 1919. One of the most well-known spiritual authors over the past several decades, Anodea Judith, has written several books that break down the characteristics of each chakra in great detail, and the types of ailments that can arise from chakra imbalances. During the New Age in the '70s, when spiritual and esoteric practices began making an appearance in the West, the chakras became more mainstream and were infused in other energy practices, such as clairvoyance, acupuncture, and, of course, Reiki. Here, in each chakra's description, you'll find information about the origins and associations of each chakra. Feel free to dive deeper into the original texts and interpretations at your will (see page 174 for more resources).

In the meantime, it is important to have a basic understanding of the characteristics of each chakra but also their ordering and progression. In the Upanishads (where chakras made their first appearance), it is suggested that energy flows up—from the Muladhara (first chakra, root) to the Sahasrara (seventh chakra, crown)—as our mind becomes purer and purer.

This actually aligns with how we develop as beings, too. Development begins at the first chakra, seated at the lowest point of the spinal column. It deals with basic survival, material needs, and our ancestry. As we age, we naturally progress to the development of higher chakras, such as love and compassion at the heart center (four).

Finally, we progress to the highest chakra (seven) at the crown of the head, where we reach connection to divinity, spirit, or whatever you like to call it.

THE ROLE OF CHAKRAS IN REIKI

While Reiki and the chakras come from two different spiritual traditions, they actually have a lot in common—it all comes back to the idea of energy (prana or ki). Many practitioners equate the tandens or hara to the chakras and realize that both systems share the idea that energy must be flowing freely through these centers for optimal overall health. In fact, there are many different ways that one can "balance" their chakras, so to speak. For example, certain yogic asanas (postures), pranayamas (breathing techniques), or physical movements can help release stuck energy and open the chakras. You can eat certain foods or listen to vibrational music to promote balance to your chakras. You can use bijas, affirmations, mantras, or deities to meditate on and heal the chakras. But one of the most beautiful ways to promote balance and restoration to the chakras is by way of Reiki healing—moving energy around in the body as needed.

When working with the chakras in Reiki, the practitioner can include a pass over each of the chakras instead of using the prescribed hands positions. The practitioner can also use a combination of hand positions to support a specific chakra. For example, if a client is experiencing challenges with trust and complains of a compressed chest, energy can specifically be offered to encourage balance to the heart chakra (more on this in chapters 9 to 15). And, not to mention, connecting the chakras to the Reiki Precepts is a great way to prepare yourself for an offering.

ROOT CHAKRA

The first chakra, *Muladhara*, is all about grounding and deals with our stability within this world. This is a Sanskrit word that translates to "root." Without a solid foundation, or rooting, it is difficult to fully grow and mature as a person. It is also difficult to progress to the higher energy states of the other chakras. As a healer, one should find grounding in the first chakra so that no insecurities or fears show up during an offering. While the idea of working with heavenly ki sounds fun, it's just as important to find stability in earth energy. Energetic issues of the first chakra can be very deep, as the development of this chakra begins in the earliest stage of our lives. It has a lasting impact on our feelings about our home, money, food, and other aspects of our environment. A deficient first chakra (lacking sufficient energy flow) for anyone can manifest in feeling disconnected from the body, out of control, or unable to settle down, while an excessive chakra (too much energy flow) can include fear of new things, rigidity, and/or hoarding of objects or food.

How each of the chakras can be balanced using Reiki will be explained in part two (see page 123).

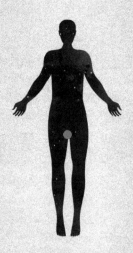

ROOT CHAKRA
MAIN CHARACTERISTICS AT A GLANCE

Sanskrit name and translation	Muladhara. "Mula" translates to "root," and "adhara" translates to "foundation" or "base"
Other names	Root support, tribal chakra
Location	Base of the spine
Correlating body parts	Excretory (rectum) and immune systems, feet and legs, bones
Color	Red
Bija	Lam
Nature Element	Earth
Physical, mental, and emotional elements to the chakra	Survival, basic needs, and primal instincts
	Center of grounding and stability, inner strength
	From where everything originates, tied to our family tree
Bringing the origin to life	According to the Upanishads, kundalini or "shakti" energy sits within the Muhladhara. Therefore, the root chakra is a great place to start to harness energy healing.
	The root chakra can be associated with the deity Ganesh, who is the "remover of obstacles." He is happy, comfortable, and well-fed. One can assimilate this narrative to remove feelings of fear, inadequacy, and insecurity tied to material matters.

SACRAL CHAKRA

The second chakra is *Svadhishthana*. Seated in the pelvis and hips and connected to our sexual organs, it is no surprise that this chakra carries much of our emotions, our movements, and our ability to be fluid. The chakra is also related to creativity. Translating to "one's own abode," it is the place or "home" within our physical and spiritual body where we express ourselves. This is why moving and dancing feel so good for the soul! As we progress as beings, it is through the second chakra that we begin to really come into ourselves and allow ourselves to partake in things and relationships (of all kinds) that give us pleasure and make us feel abundant. A deficiency in the second chakra can appear as someone who denies themselves pleasures or has too many boundaries. An excessive second chakra would be someone on the opposite spectrum—someone who may have poor boundaries or indulges a little too much.

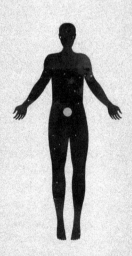

SACRAL CHAKRA
MAIN CHARACTERISTICS AT A GLANCE

Sanskrit name and translation	Svadhishthana, which translates to "one's own abode"
Other names	Sacred home, special, or sweet abode
Location	Hips and pelvis
Correlating body parts	Reproductive and sex organs, excretory system (bladder), large intestine
Color	Orange
Bija	Vam
Element	Water
Physical, mental, and emotional elements to the chakra	Movement and sexuality, emotional regulation From where desires, pleasures, and creativity originate Allows us to be fluid and adaptable human beings
Bringing the origin to life	In the lotus of the sacral chakra sits a crocodile-like animal who harnesses kundalini energy. In order to keep moving up the spiritual path, he satisfies his desires and passions. We can incorporate this practice by allowing ourselves the freedom to create, to enjoy, and to explore our passions.

SOLAR PLEXUS CHAKRA

The third chakra is *Manipura*, and it is the space where we find our personal power and begin to form our identity. Picture a *mani* (the Sanskrit word for "gem") in the pit of your belly. Ideally, the gem should be shining brightly like the sun, but many fears or insecurities can dim this light and inhibit us from pursuing our dreams. It makes sense that our third chakra is connected to our gut. Gut feelings—arguably just as important, if not more important, than our thoughts—may either propel us forward or hold us back. The third chakra is also known as the center of transformation, because heat and fire are often required for change, both physically and metaphorically. It is important to think about the progression of the lower chakras to the third chakra here. A strong foundation, coupled with our passions and desires, should give us the will to take actions that are important to us in the third chakra. Therefore, a deficiency in the third chakra ends up with someone feeling fatigued and having poor self-discipline and low self-esteem. An excessive third chakra could look like someone who is egocentric, aggressive, and/or too authoritative.

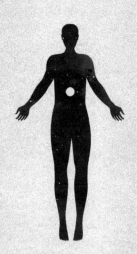

SOLAR PLEXUS CHAKRA
MAIN CHARACTERISTICS AT A GLANCE

Sanskrit name and translation	Manipura. "Mani" translates to "jewel," and "pura" to "city," or "the city of jewels"
Other names	Power center, lustrous gem
Location	Navel
Correlating body parts	Digestive organs, abdomen, kidneys, adrenal glands
Color	Yellow
Bija	Ram
Element	Fire
Physical, mental, and emotional elements to the chakra	Energy and metabolism The center of transformation Source of power and willpower, autonomy, and overcoming fears
Bringing the origin to life	This chakra is associated with Agni, the god of fire, which is why when we think of a strong third chakra, it's all about igniting that fire or taking some sort of action.

HEART CHAKRA

Next on this path is the fourth chakra, *Anahata*. There is
no doubt that this is one of the most special places in our
spiritual body—our heart center! The midway between
the body and the spirit. It translates to "unhurt," but metaphorically it means the ability to be unshaken and have
no hurt in the heart, despite past hurtful experiences. It
is the ability to have unconditional love and compassion
for ourselves and one another, to be living in peace and
harmony, and to use our power established earlier for
goodness. This is also an important chakra for any healer,
as one should be kind to themselves and others during an
offering, and lead with an open heart, just like the Reiki
Precept says. Deficiency in the heart chakra can manifest
in feeling lonely or depressed, having a poor connection
to others, or having a hard time trusting anyone. An
excessive fourth chakra could make someone too giving
or too trusting.

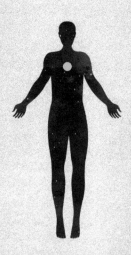

HEART CHAKRA
MAIN CHARACTERISTICS AT A GLANCE

Sanskrit name	*Anahata*, which translates to "unhurt" or "pure"
Other names	None
Location	Heart center
Correlating body parts	Cardiovascular, respiratory and circulatory systems, shoulders, arms and hands, ribs, breasts
Color	Green
Bija	Yam
Element	Air
Physical, mental, and emotional elements to the chakra	Feelings of unconditional love and compassion, peace and bliss Center of relationships Where we find balance, healing, and unity
Bringing the origin to life	In the Upanishads, it is said that when the mind becomes more purified, it rises to the Anahata chakra, where one can begin to experience true bliss. One of the deities most associated with the heart chakra is Krishna, the god of love and compassion. Tied to bhakti yoga (Krishna), or the yoga of service, a part of our spiritual journey should be to find compassion toward ourselves and others.

THROAT CHAKRA

The fifth chakra is *Vishuddha*, meaning "to purify," and it is located in our throat. It allows us to communicate with others and the world—to speak our truth, essentially. It also allows us to interpret sounds, vibrations, and words. There is a component of self-expression and creativity at this chakra. A person with a deficient fifth chakra could have difficulty expressing themselves, or may be afraid to speak up or share. Someone who has an excessive fifth chakra may talk too much without enough listening.

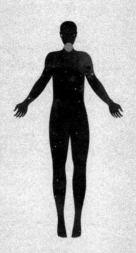

THROAT CHAKRA
MAIN CHARACTERISTICS AT A GLANCE

Sanskrit name and translation	Vishuddha, which translates to "to purify"
Other names	Seat of responsibility
Location	Throat
Correlating body parts	Neck, thyroid, larynx, mouth, hypothalamus
Color	Turquoise or blue
Bija	Ham
Element	Aether
Physical, mental, and emotional elements to the chakra	Center of communication Relates to sound and vibrations Speaking your truth and self-expression, consent
Bringing the origin to life	The representation of this chakra is a silver crescent, the lunar symbol of cosmic sound. Beyond the obvious communication, it is representative of us living in vibrational harmony. Inherent to the name of this chakra, to reach this level one must be purified in the lower chakras.

THIRD EYE CHAKRA

The sixth chakra is *Ajna*, and you've probably heard it referenced in a yoga or meditation class a million times, since it's also known as the third eye. Our third eye is in charge of *inner* sight, or inner knowing, so this chakra is highly mental. Thus, our ability to be intuitive, our ability to make "the right" or "better" choice, can depend on the health of our sixth chakra. Don't we all just want to know where to go next? Whether the path we are on, or about to embark on, is truly for us? But to level to this point requires patience, maturity, and a strong awareness of our self, which we saw and built on in the earlier chakras. It is also interesting that the Sanskrit word Ajna can literally mean "to perceive" or "to command." So it is about not only our perceptions, but also our ability to take our perceptions and know how to integrate them into reality. A deficient sixth chakra includes the inability to visualize, poor decision-making, poor imagination, or even poor memory. An excessive sixth chakra can mean being too delusional, obsessive, or not in control.

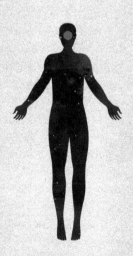

THIRD EYE CHAKRA
MAIN CHARACTERISTICS AT A GLANCE

Sanskrit name	Ajna, which translates to "to command" or "to perceive"
Other names	Third eye, command center
Location	The space between the two eyebrows
Correlating body parts	Brain, pineal gland, nervous system, eyes, nose, and ears
Color	Indigo
Bija	Om
Element	Some say thought, while others say none, as when this chakra is reached, the level is beyond the physical elements
Physical, mental, and emotional elements to the chakra	How we process symbols and signals in reality Center of intuition, inner knowing, imagination, and vision Considered the seat of the mind
Bringing the origin to life	The third eye chakra is the point at which the major Ida and the Pingala nadis (or energy channels) cross before reaching the crown chakra. In the Upanishads, this is one of the highest energetic states, where one begins to connect to the supreme self or Brahman.

CROWN CHAKRA

Finally, the seventh chakra is *Sahasrara*, which means "thousand-petaled lotus." This is the top shelf of the chakra system at the crown of the head, the place where one begins to transcend earthly matters. The number 1,000 is a very sacred number in the yogic tradition, indicating infinity. Whereas the sixth chakra is more about inner sight, the knowing here in the seventh chakra comes from a divine source. It is also what allows us the power to manifest. Therefore, the energy of this chakra can be very intense yet very important and influential for healing issues of the lower chakras. Connecting to the energy of the crown chakra can also allow one a great sense of relief. It is like the white light that shines down upon us and keeps us sane in everyday life! Deficiencies here may appear as an inability or lack of desire to connect to spirit or too much emphasis on matters of the lower chakras (material things). Excesses could be an inability to "come down" from a spiritual high (to come back to Earth) or confusion.

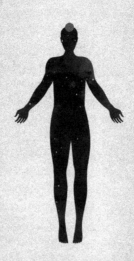

CROWN CHAKRA
MAIN CHARACTERISTICS AT A GLANCE

Sanskrit name and translation	Sahasrara, translates to "infinity," "thousand," or "thousand-petaled lotus"
Other names	None
Location	The crown of the head
Correlating body parts	Pituitary gland
Color	Violet
Bija	None
Element	Some say thought, while others say none, as when this chakra is reached, the level is beyond the physical elements
Physical, mental, and emotional elements to the chakra	Consciousness and thought Transcendence, enlightenment, our higher self Center of divinity, connection to the divine source and other spiritual beings
Bringing the origin to life	Considered "Avastha" (the highest state in Sanskrit), this is the point at which one really becomes one with Brahman, God, or spirit. It is the highest place of consciousness and the highest place where kundalini energy rises.

SEVEN CHAKRAS VS. FIVE ELEMENTS OF REIKI

As explained previously in the history of Reiki, this practice comes from Buddhism, which means that before the chakras were incorporated, the practice reflected the five elements philosophy from Japanese Buddhism: Earth, Water, Fire, Wind, and Void (Aether).

The Reiki mantras reflect these elements in their sounds. Choku Rei, the mantra for the first symbol, and linked to earth energy, has more Earth element sounds, while Sei Heki, the mantra for the second symbol and linked to heavenly energy, has more fire element sounds.

Taking a closer look, we realize the five elements and chakras share the same principle: They point the way toward areas that require balance. However, the chakras are located in specific parts of our body, while the Japanese elements can encompass the area of multiple chakras. The Earth element, for example, would encompass chakras 1, 2, and 3. Also, one chakra can have qualities from more than an element. For example, chakra 2 has qualities from the Earth and water elements.

EARTH. This element represents the objects of Earth, like stones in nature, or bones in people. Emotionally, it is associated with rigidity, collectiveness, stability, physicality, and gravity.
Chakras: 1, 2, 3.

WATER. The element of water is associated with fluid, flowing, and formless things—like rivers or our bloodstream. The qualities represented by this element are emotion, defensiveness, adaptability, flexibility, suppleness, and charisma.
Chakras: 2, 4.

FIRE. Fire is linked to the energetic, forceful, moving things in the world, like animals and body heat. It also represents drive, passion, security, motivation, intention, and extroversion.

Chakras: 3.

WIND. Wind is related to all the things that grow, expand, and have freedom of movement—like air, smoke, and knowledge. It is also associated with breathing, evasiveness, benevolence, compassion, and wisdom.

Chakras: 4.

VOID (AETHER). This element represents things beyond our everyday experience, particularly those made of pure energy, like spirit, thought, creativity, and communication. It is also associated with power, spontaneity, inventiveness, and the concept of "emptiness" in Buddhism (interconnection).

Chakras: 5, 6, 7.

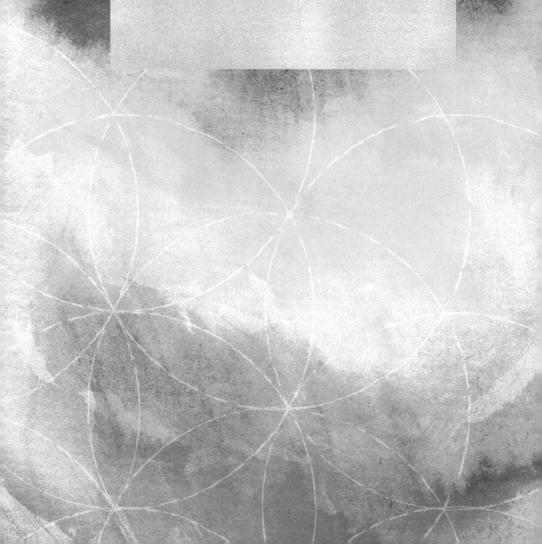

CHAPTER 6

REIKI SYMBOLS

The Reiki symbols have a sacred nature. Working with them allows you to connect to primordial energies, let go of layers of conditioning, and increase your energy flow. You may come across different versions of the symbol. This is because when Hawayo Takata taught the masters who originated most of the current Reiki lineages, she didn't allow them to take notes during class. Slight variations were then introduced. It is best to draw the symbol the way you were taught, as you already have a connection with it.

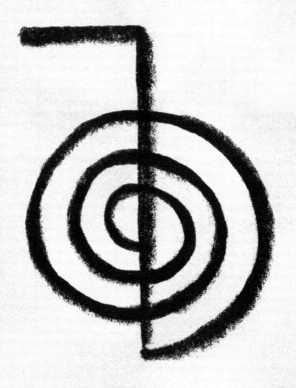

CHOKU REI (POWER)

The first symbol, associated with the mantra Choku Rei (pronounced cho-koo-ray), is known as the Power symbol or CKR. That is because Choku Rei can be translated from Japanese as "place the power of the universe here."

In many Reiki styles, this translation has been applied literally, and CKR is used to increase energy or power-up other symbols. In its inception, though, "place the power of the universe here" was meant as a reminder that "you hold the power of the universe inside yourself." Hence the inward spiral that composes most of the symbol.

CKR is associated with earth energy (grounding) and the quality of focus. If we remember that energy follows the mind, we can see how a capacity for focus will increase the power of your energy. Working with CKR allows you to:

- Be more grounded, focused, and centered

- Feel safe and protected

- Hold more energy

- Clear your vision, take things less personally

- Pick up less "vibes" from other people (a lifesaver for empaths!)

HOW TO WORK WITH CKR:

- Draw it in front of you with the palm of your hand or with your eyes. Activate it by repeating its mantra three times (aloud or in your head), and step into the energetic space you created.

- Visualize it inside in your body during meditation.

- Chant its mantra as meditation (see sidebar, page 70), or silently in your head during sessions if you are feeling a bit dizzy or distracted.

- Some Reiki lineages draw CKR on all the chakras (front and back of the body) and palms to open and close Reiki sessions. This helps the practitioner focus and get into the right state of mind to offer treatment.

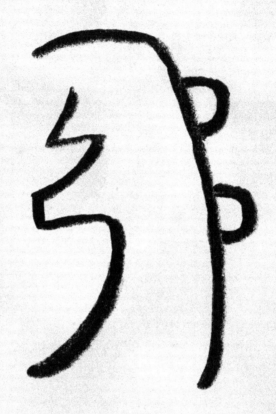

SEI HEKI (HARMONY)

The second symbol, associated with the mantra Sei Heki (pronounced say-hay-kee), is known as the Harmony symbol or SHK. Sei Heki can be translated as "mental habit" and is often used to help manage addictions. However, the mental habit the symbol refers to is the one of seeing ourselves as separate from the universe and every living being.

It is associated with heavenly energy, spiritual connection, psychic ability, and vision. Working with SHK allows you to:

- Increase your intuition and psychic abilities

- Let go of limiting beliefs

- Reduce emotional resistance

- Spark creativity

- Soften physical tension and emotional and mental rigidity

HOW TO WORK WITH SHK:

- Draw it in front of you with the palm of your hand or with your eyes. Activate it by repeating its mantra three times, and step into the energetic space you created.

- Visualize it inside your body during meditation.

- Chant its mantra as meditation (see sidebar, page 70), or silently in your head during sessions to strengthen the connection to your intuition.

- Some Reiki lineages activate SHK by bookending it with CKR (you draw and activate CKR, then SHK, then CKR again). In other lineages, you work directly with SHK. Just be sure to balance this high-vibrating energy with grounding modalities, so you don't feel spacey, or become too emotional or forgetful.

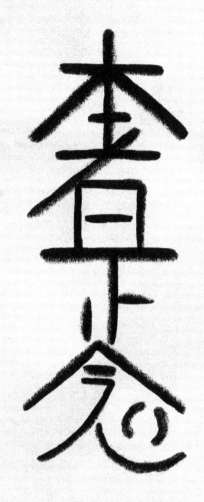

HON SHA ZE SHO NEN (DISTANCE)

The third symbol, associated with the mantra Hon Sha Ze Sho Nen (pronounced hon-shaw-ze-show-nen), is known as the Distance symbol or HSZSN. This symbol is the combination of five Japanese characters and can be translated as "my original nature is correct thought." "Correct thought" refers to oneness or nonduality.

HSZSN is associated with the heart center, reminding us that we are interconnected to every living being and everything in the universe. Working with this symbol allows you to create a space where and time and distance do not exist, so you can:

- Do remote Reiki sessions for people who need it (see the "how to" in chapter 7, page 103)

- Hold a healing space for the whole planet

- Offer Reiki treatments to animals you can't touch

- Help heal the past and ancestral traumas

HOW TO WORK WITH HSZSN:

- Draw it in the air. Activate it by repeating its mantra three times, and step into the energetic space you created.

- Draw it on paper; place your hand on the symbol; and activate it by repeating the mantra three times and feel its energy.

- Chant its mantra as meditation (see sidebar, page 70), or silently in your head during sessions when you want to increase your connection with your client.

- Some Reiki lineages activate HSZSN by book-ending it with CKR (you draw and activate CKR, then HSZSN, then CKR again). In other lineages, you work directly with HSZSN. They are just different ways of connecting consciously with beautiful heart energy.

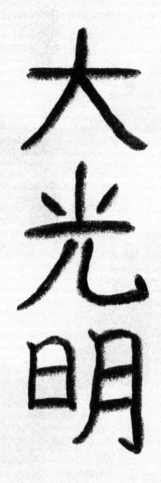

DAI KOMYO (MASTER)

While the other three symbols and mantras are learned in the second level, the fourth symbol is taught during Level 3. It is associated with the mantra Dai Komyo (pronounced dye-ko-mee-o), which is known as the Master symbol or DKM. This symbol consists of three Japanese characters and can be translated as "big, bright light." It represents the pure light of our true nature and the state of enlightenment.

If the Reiki symbols were a tree, CKR would be the roots; SHK, the foliage; HSZSN, the trunk; and DKM would be the light that surrounds and feeds the whole tree—because it is symbolic of the source from where everything comes. DKM encompasses the energies of all symbols—on steroids. Working with this symbol allows you to create a space of oneness to:

- Perform attunements

- Increase the flow of energy

- Release deep layers of conditioning

- Balance all energies

HOW TO WORK WITH DKM:

- Draw it in the air. Activate it by repeating its mantra three times, and step into it, and let it fill you with its beautiful energy like a waterfall.

- Draw it during attunements.

- Chant its mantra as a meditation (see sidebar, page 70) or silently in your head during attunements to stay in the space of oneness.

- Use it for remote sessions instead of HSZSN.

When starting to work with DKM, do so sparingly to avoid feeling too spacey. You can counterbalance it with lots of meditations with CKR to keep grounded.

REIKI MANTRAS

Each Reiki symbol has a correlating mantra that is often used as its name. Although these mantras are commonly used in conjunction with the symbols to activate their power, you can work with them on their own to boost your connection to different types of energies.

One of the most powerful ways to work with the mantras is through chanting. Our bodies are made of approximately 60 percent water. Specifically, our brain and heart are composed of up to 73 percent of this element. When we chant, the sound travels through the water. This vibration helps balance the energy in your whole body. Chanting also makes your thoracic cavity vibrate. Most organs are stored there. The vibration relaxes your organs and helps them release tension and toxins. You can chant the full mantra or use the shortened versions below:

Choku Rei ——— o-u-e-i (pronounced o-oo-way-ee)

Sei Heki ——— e-i-e-ki (pronounced ay-ee-ay-kee)

Hon Sha Ze Sho Nen ——— o-a-ze-o-ne (pronounced o-ah-zay-o-nay)

Dai Komyo ——— a-i-ko-yo (pronounced eye-ee-ko-yo)

Always chant one mantra at a time. Here is how:

1. Set the intention to receive the healing needed in the moment.

2. Take a deep breath from the hara (lower belly).

3. Chant the mantra one, two, or three times depending on your lung capacity.

4. Make sure you finish the mantra in the same breath—better to chant only one full mantra per breath than breaking one in the middle.

5. Make sure to shape the sounds clearly using your lips.

6. After you are done chanting, sit with your eyes closed, feeling the resonance and the energetic space you created.

CHAPTER 7

HAND POSITIONS

We often think of hands-on healing as something magical. But In reality, it is innate to all humans. A mother's first reaction to soothe her child is to use touch. So, when it comes to performing hands-on healing, we invite you to approach it as an act of reconnecting with your body, your spirit, and your energy. As an act of surrender, setting the intention to receive the healing needed during the session.

And when in doubt, use the Reiki Precepts to guide you: Try to get the hands in the right position, but do not worry. Remember that presence, compassion, and loving-kindness are more important than being exact. Also, we all have different body shapes and sizes, so feel free to adapt these positions to a way that feels comfortable to you.

SELF-HEALING

Before getting into the hand positions, here is a short protocol you can use for your session:

- Start with three deep breaths into your lower belly (hara) to center yourself.

- If you work with symbols, chant them silently in your head (three times each).

- Perform Gassho to set your intention to receive the healing needed during the session (you can also meditate in Gassho for a few minutes).

- All the way through the hand positions, try to keep your thumbs tucked along with your hands, and your hands slightly cupped and fingers together.

- If you get distracted, take a deep breath all the way down to your lower belly and exhale, letting the energy flow through your hands.

- In time, start using your intuition to come up with your own set of hand positions.

- When finished, place your hands in Gassho to express gratitude for the healing received.

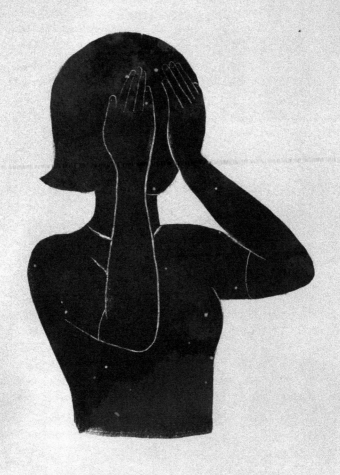

Eyes

Gently cup your hands over your eyes, without touching them. The palms should be over your eyes, the heels of your hands placed along each cheekbone, and your fingertips on the top of your forehead.

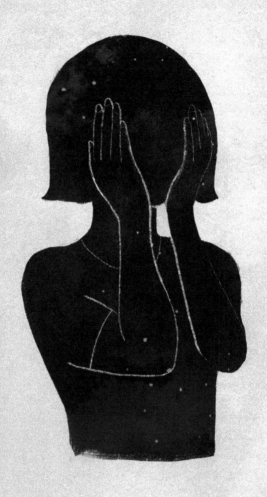

Ears

Cup your hands over your ears. The palms should cover your ears, the heels of your hands placed along your jaw, and your fingertips resting lightly on your temples.

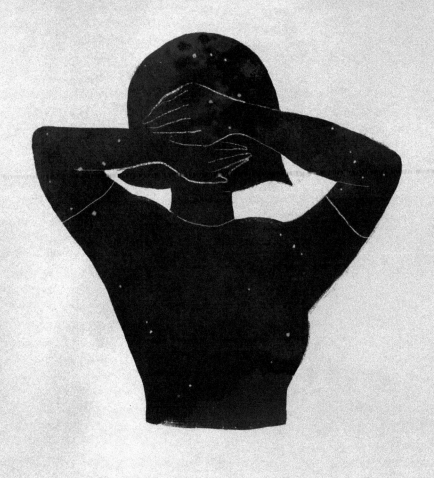

Back of the head

Place both hands on the back of your head, stacked one above the other. (It doesn't matter which one is above or below.) Fingertips should point horizontally. The lower hand should be cupping the back of your skull.

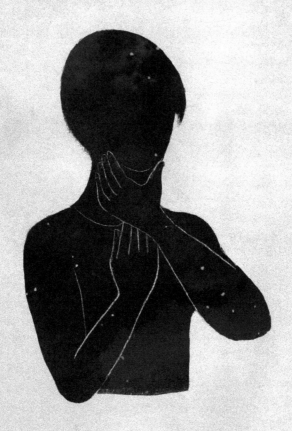

Throat and heart

Place your left hand diagonally across your throat, with its heel on your left collarbone and the fingertips on your right jaw. Place the right hand horizontally on the heart area, at the center of your chest. The left hand can rest on the right hand.

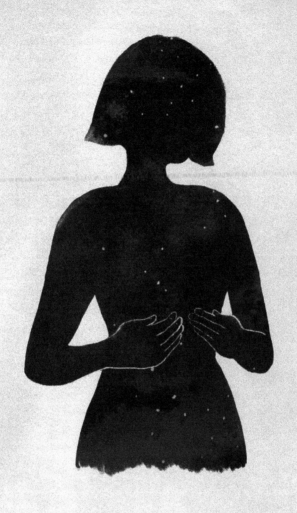

Solar plexus

With your arms parallel to the floor, place your hands just below your chest or breasts, with the fingertips together along the bottom of your sternum and the heels touching your rib cage on each side.

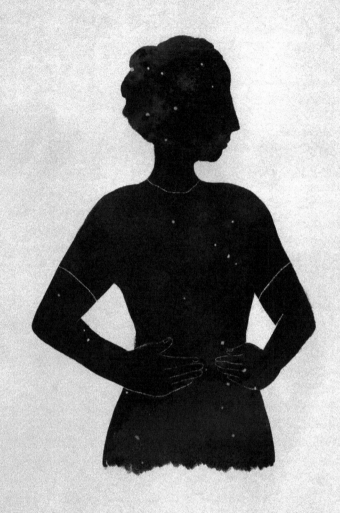

Abdomen

Place each middle finger on your belly button, and cup your hands over your abdominal region.

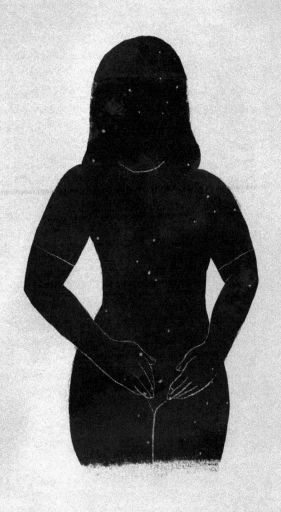

Groin

Place the heels of your hands where your legs meet your abdomen, and place your fingertips along the inner thighs.

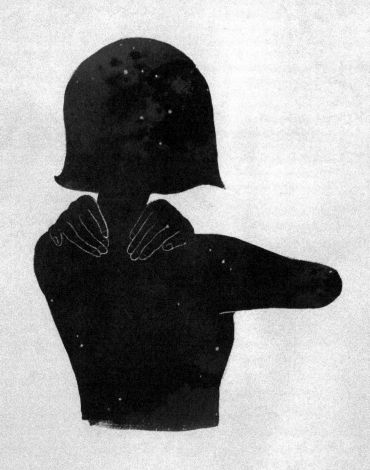

Shoulders

With your arms either crossed or uncrossed, rest the heels of your hands on your collarbones, and cup your shoulders. Your fingertips should rest on the backs of your shoulders.

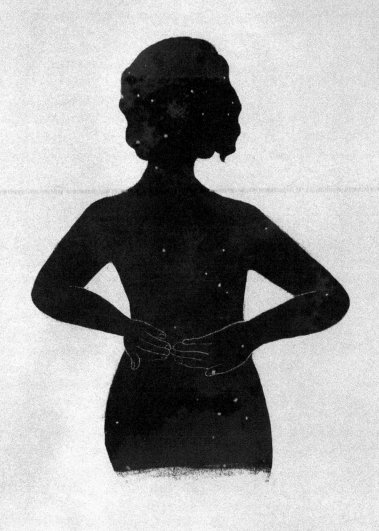

Middle back

Bend your elbows and place the heels of your hands on either side of your rib cage. Cup your hands over your back (at the height of the kidneys), fingers pointing to the spine.

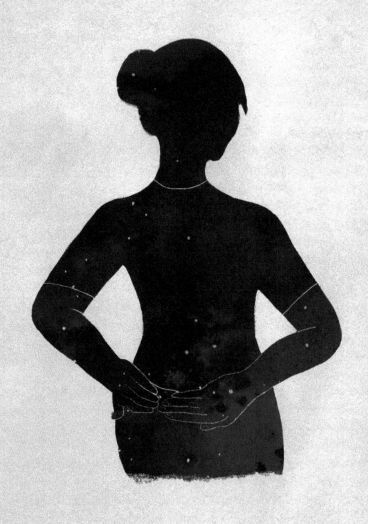

Lower back

With the heels of your hands along your sides above your hips, point your fingers toward your spine, letting them rest on top of your pelvic bone.

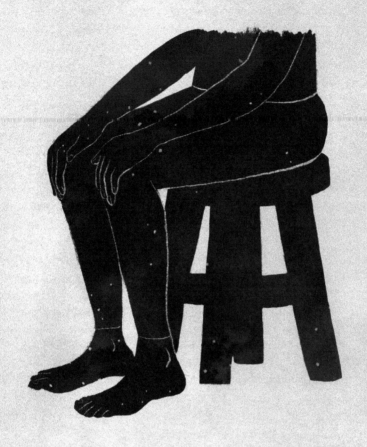

Knees

Cover each knee with one hand, with the heels on top and the fingers curved down over the kneecap.

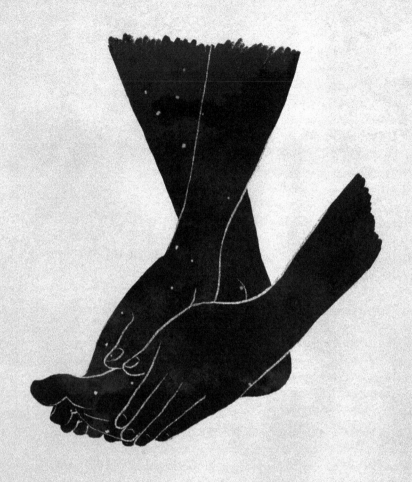

Feet

One foot at a time, cup one hand over the bottom of the foot, and the other hand over the top.

HEALING OTHERS

The protocol to share a hands-on healing session with another person is the same as the one for self-care, except for the intention. You can make it very specific: "May (name of the recipient) receive the healing needed," or less specific: "May we and all living beings receive the healing needed during this session." Choose what feels right.

While offering a session to another, remember: You are not doing the healing, you are facilitating it. Just be present, hold the space compassionately, and let the energy flow.

During the session, try to keep your spine straight, arms relaxed, and eyes open to stay grounded. If you feel dizzy or drained, you may need grounding. Doing deep belly breathing or meditating with the first symbol can help.

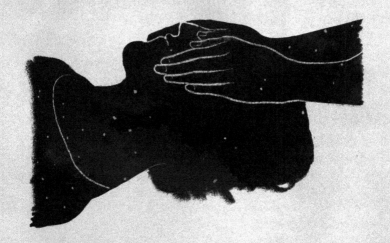

Eyes

Stand or sit at the crown of the person. Place the heels of both hands on the hairline, and cup your hands over the eyes. Rest your fingertips lightly on the cheekbones.

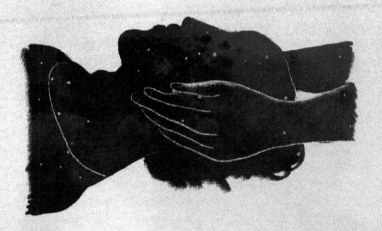

Ears

Cup your hands over the person's ears, with the heels resting gently on the temples and the fingertips pointing downward to the body.

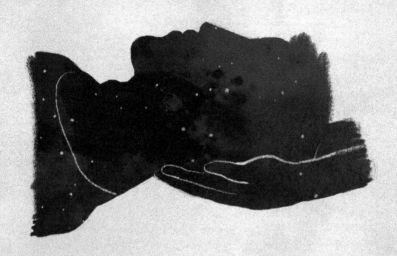

Back of the head

Slide your hands under the person's head. Your finger-tips should be along the occipital bone, and the heels of your hands along the top of the head. Try to keep the pinkies together.

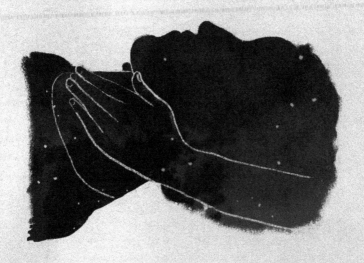

Throat

Place the heels of your hands gently on the jawbone or collarbone (where it meets the shoulders) and cup your hands over the throat. Avoid touching the throat directly—it is a very sensitive area and can make your client uncomfortable.

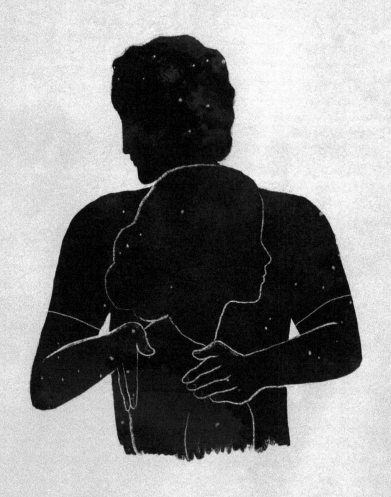

Heart

Move to the side of the person. Place one hand along the sternum (just above the chest) and the other one along the collarbone. If offering treatment to a female, be careful to avoid the breasts.

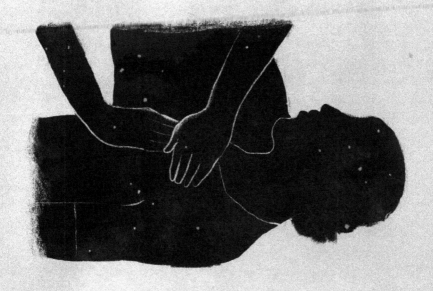

Solar plexus

Line up one hand in front of the other (fingertips from one hand touching the heel of the other hand), and place them on the rib cage, just below the chest.

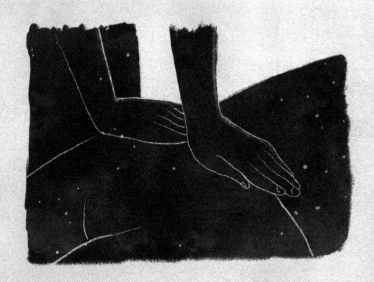

Navel

Keep your hands in the same alignment. (You can switch which one goes in front to relieve tension in the shoulders.) Place them at the level of the belly button. Ask the person to point to the belly button if needed.

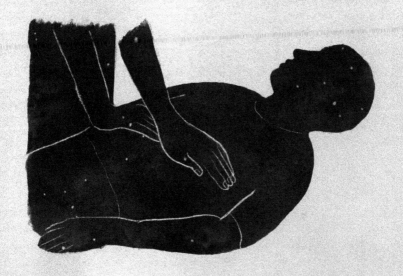

Hara

Same position as the navel, just one hand-width lower.

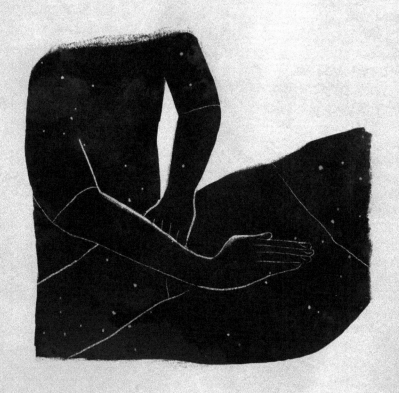

Groin

Place the heel of one hand on the top crease of one side of the hip bone, and cup it diagonally alongside the top of the leg toward the inner crease. Place the other heel on the inner crease of the hip, and cup the hand all the way to the outer crease of the other side.

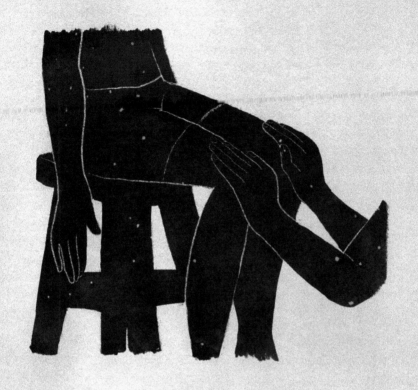

Knees

Cover one knee with each hand.

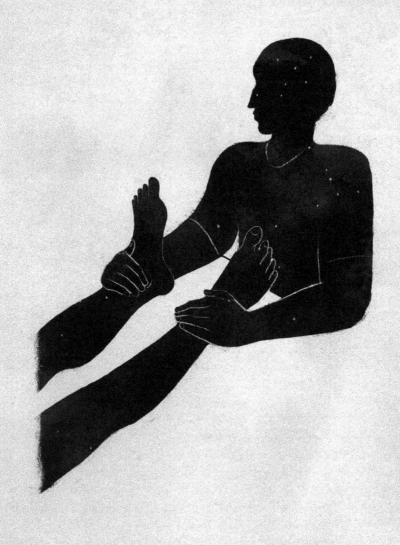

Ankles

Move to the person's feet. Place the heel of each hand on the outer sides of the ankles. Wrap your hands over the ankles, with the fingertips resting on the inner sides.

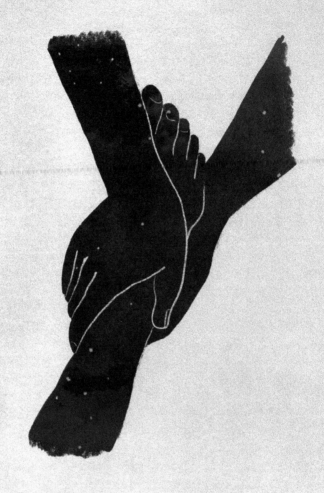

Feet

One foot at a time, hold the arch with one hand and cover the top of the foot with the other.

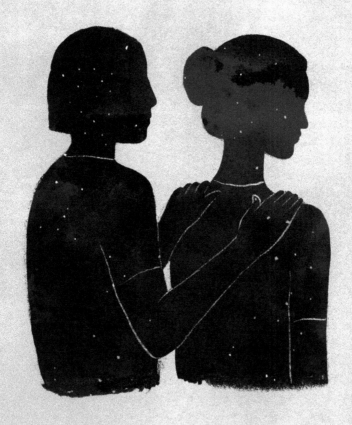

Shoulders

Standing to one side, place your hands (one in front of the other) across the back of the shoulders.

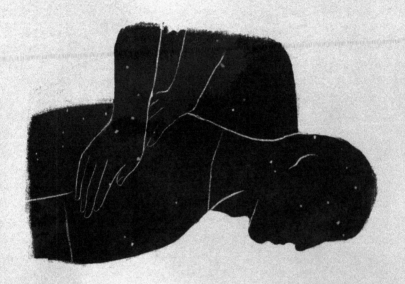

Middle back

Keeping the same position (as for Shoulders), move your hands approximately one hand-width lower.

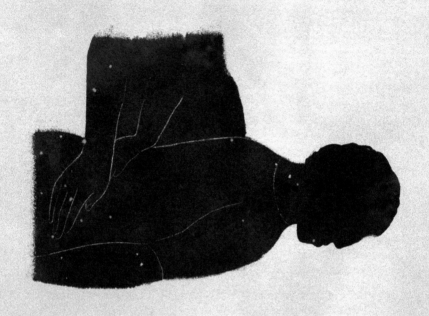

Lower back

Move your hands to the lower back, at about waist level.

DISTANCE HEALING

Remote or distance healing is traditionally taught in Reiki 2, the level in which you learn the Distance symbol (HSZSN). By working with this symbol, we remember that we are all interconnected and enter an energetic space where geographical location is no longer relevant. There are many ways to offer distance Reiki sessions. We invite you to try them all and choose the one that feels best for you.

DISTANCE REIKI METHOD #1

For this surrogate method, as well as all distance reiki sessions, ask for the person's full name and location and, if possible, a photo—so you can picture the recipient in your mind. Schedule a time in advance. Contact the recipient before starting so the person can get comfortable and set the intention to receive the healing needed. You can also text at the end to let the recipient know the session is over.

Using yourself as a surrogate:

1. Take three deep breaths into your lower belly to center yourself.

2. Draw HSZSN and repeat its mantra three times to activate it. You can also visualize it or chant the mantra for a few minutes. Some lineages draw CKR first, then HSZSN, and then CKR to help focus the energy.

3. Perform Gassho to set your intention of sharing the healing needed for [name] in [city and country]. Look at the photo if available.

4. Perform the hand positions for the self.

5. Close with Gassho to give thanks.

Using an object:

Follow the same protocol but, instead of your body, use a plush toy, a doll, or a pillow.

Use your hands to cover whole areas of the toy or doll: head, shoulders, torso, hips, legs.

When working with a pillow, imagine the top is the head and the bottom, the feet.

DISTANCE REIKI METHOD #2

This method is pretty effective and easy to do as well:

1. If you have a photo of the person, print it. If you don't have one, skip to the next step.

2. Write the name and location on a paper or the photo printout.

3. Place it between your hands.

4. Take three deep breaths to center yourself.

5. Draw or visualize HSZSN for a few minutes.

6. Set the intention to share the healing with the recipient.

7. Let the energy flow between your hands for 10 to 15 minutes.

8. Close with Gassho to give thanks.

This method is the simplest and, because of that, sometimes the hardest to keep focused: Simply hold the person in your mind and heart.

1. Take three deep breaths into your lower belly to center yourself.

2. Draw or visualize HSZSN for a few minutes.

3. Place your hands in Gassho to set your intention to share the healing needed.

4. Hold that person in your mind and heart while you let the energy flow. Do this for 10 to 15 minutes. You can also imagine them sitting in front of you, and let the energy flow.

5. Close with Gassho to give thanks.

REIKI FOR PETS AND PLANTS

As mentioned in chapter 1 (see page 4), everything in the universe has ki. This means your Reiki practice can go beyond people to include your pets or plants. Try it. They will love it and benefit from it greatly in terms of calmness, energy levels, and overall health.

Here are a few tips on sharing Reiki with pets:

- Forget about determined hand positions. If the animal likes touch, just set the intention for it to receive the healing needed and let the energy flow as you pet it. You may witness your pet wiggling around to place certain body parts under your hands.

- Cats seldom like touch. Just point your hands toward them and visualize the energy flowing to them. You can draw or chant the Distance symbol and mantra (HSZSN) to strengthen the connection.

- For animals you shouldn't touch or who won't let themselves be touched, follow the distance protocol. You can also use a surrogate if it makes it easier for you. (Some people like to use plush animals or pillows.)

- Keep the sessions short (five to 15 minutes). Animals don't have mental barriers toward energy work, which means they are very sensitive to Reiki. If the animal moves away, don't take it personally: This is their way to tell you they have had enough.

How to share Reiki with plants:

- Place your hands on the plant's container and let the energy flow for three to five minutes. While you do this, feel the connection with the plant.

- Scan the plant with your hands, and let them hover over the parts on which you feel a sensation (pulling, tingling, warmth, cold). Keep them there for a minute or two and then scan again. You can do this for 10 minutes.

- Place your hands on the watering can or the plant's food, and let the energy flow. Then water and feed the plant.

After a few short sessions, you will notice your plants may grow faster and taller than usual and look perkier!

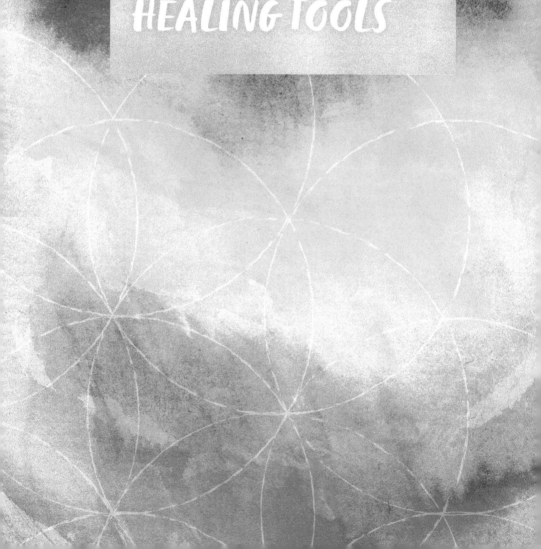

CHAPTER 8

COMPLEMENTARY HEALING TOOLS

There are many complementary natural healing tools you can use alongside your Reiki practice, which can boost the healing process and create a pleasant environment. Try incorporating one or two of these at a time, and see which ones resonate with you most. Each of the tools in this chapter can also be tied to whatever chakra or type of energy you might be targeting on a given day.

CRYSTALS

Crystals, minerals, and other stones (referred to as crystals to keep it simple) can absorb, hold, and radiate energy, which is why some practitioners like to use them during Reiki sessions to magnify the healing. Crystals are also associated with the chakras based on their color, element, and physical and metaphysical qualities.

To work with crystals, you can either place them on the person receiving treatment or create a crystal grid right next to them—for example, under the table or chair. If placed on the person, make sure they feel comfortable (that the crystals are not too heavy, too hot, or too cold). Also, make sure you clear or cleanse the crystals before and after use (for example, by sunlight, moonlight, smudge, tap water, or saltwater). You can also open and close the Reiki session by drawing the symbol, if you are working with one, over each crystal, or over the cleansing water you'll ultimately use to clean the crystals at the end. This is to make sure they do not carry any energy with them that may have been absorbed during the session.

There are two ways you can choose the crystals for the session. The first way is more intuitive and interactive for the person you are performing Reiki on. From your collection of crystals, allow the person receiving treatment to pick the ones that are most appealing to them. Then, use your knowledge of the chakras to place the crystals on their body over each chakra accordingly. Alternatively, the practitioner can choose the stones based on the chakra or intention the person wants to work on.

There are hundreds of different crystals that can be used for healing. Below are a few recommended crystals for each chakra.

ROOT: Garnet, Obsidian, Pyrite

SACRAL: Carnelian, Tiger's Eye, Amber

SOLAR PLEXUS: Citrine, Golden Calcite, Goldstone

HEART: Green Aventurine, Rose Quartz, Green Tourmaline

THROAT: Aquamarine, Angelite, Topaz

THIRD EYE: Lapis Lazuli, Iolite, Kyanite

CROWN: Selenite, Amethyst, Clear Quartz

ESSENTIAL OILS

Scents and aromas have been used since the beginning of time to promote good energy and ward off disease. Essential oils can be applied either to the practitioner's wrists or temples or on others' temples. (Be sure to ask for permission first!) You can also put a couple of drops of the oils into a diffuser and let it run during the session. Most people find essential oils to be pleasant, but some people are sensitive to certain smells, and smells can also be tied to memories. It's best to ask before a session if it's okay to use them, and let the person know what scent you're planning to use. Here are some recommendations for targeting specific chakras.

Root: Earthy or herbaceous aromas such as patchouli, rosemary, or frankincense promote grounding during a session.

Sacral: Playful or spicy aromas such as sweet orange or cardamom invite a sense of invigoration.

Solar Plexus: Energizing oils such as peppermint or tea tree promote awakening and the release of sluggish energy. Peppermint is also great for promoting healthy digestion.

Heart: Rose oil and other florals are associated with love and great for connecting with the heart space.

Throat: Tea tree and eucalyptus oils have a menthol-like scent and are great for opening the nasal passages. Sage oil helps treat thyroid disorders.

Third Eye: Lavender oil is great for reducing anxiety and calming the nervous system. Chamomile is another soothing and calming oil.

Crown: Both frankincense and sandalwood oils are associated with meditation, prayer, and holiness.

MEDITATION

There are several Reiki-specific meditations you can use to stimulate the hara and balance energy.

Kenyoku Ho. This is a practice used to clear the meridians. You can use it before and after sessions.

1. Place your right hand on your left shoulder. Inhale, and on the exhale, sweep your right hand from your left shoulder down your chest toward the right hip.

2. Move to the other side. Inhale, and on the exhale, sweep your left hand from your right shoulder down your chest toward your left hip.

3. Repeat step 1.

4. With the left elbow against your side and your right arm perpendicular to the ground, place your right hand on the left shoulder. Inhale and exhale as you sweep downward toward the left fingertips.

5. Move to the other side. With the right elbow against your side and your left arm perpendicular to the ground, place your left hand on the right shoulder. Inhale and exhale as you sweep downward toward the right fingertips.

6. Repeat step 4.

7. Place your hands in Gassho.

Joshin Kokyu Ho. This meditation is used to focus the mind, clear the meridians, and build energy in the hara.

1. Find a comfortable seat.

2. Close your eyes and place your hands on your thighs with the palms facing up.

3. Inhale and feel the energy coming in through the nose and moving down to the hara.

4. Pause, feeling the energy fill your whole being.

5. Exhale to send all of the energy completely out of the body.

6. Repeat as many times as you wish and close with Gassho.

Seishin Toitsu. Seishin translates to "pure mind" and Toitsu to "gathering together." This is a meditation for alignment. We align our breath and mind, spirit and body, and heart and hara.

1. Place your hands in Gassho and focus on the hara.

2. Inhale to draw energy into your hands as it moves up to the arms and down through your body into the hara.

3. Exhale to visualize energy moving from the hara back up through the body, through the arms and out through the hands.

4. Repeat as many times as you wish.

Hatsurei Ho. Translated as "to bring forth" (Hatsu), "spirit" (Rei), and "method" (Ho), this is a meditation that includes Gassho, reciting the Precepts, Kenyoku Ho, Joshin Kokyu Ho, and Seishin Toitsu in that order. It is used to bring forth your spiritual abilities and prepare you for Reiki practice.

Meditations with symbols. As explained back in chapter 6 (see page 61), you can meditate with each of the Reiki symbols by drawing the symbol, visualizing the symbol, and chanting the symbol's mantra.

- Choku Rei for grounding (chakras 1, 2, and 3)
- Hon Sha Ze Sho Nen (chakra 4)
- Sei Heki (chakras 5, 6, and 7)

MUSIC

Music is encouraged to promote peace and relaxation during a Reiki session. Here are some ideas and considerations.

Choose music that does not include any vocals. Lyrics can be distracting for the person receiving the session. Speaking of distractions, if you are using your phone to play the music, make sure you turn it on silent or do not disturb mode, so notifications do not cause a distraction.

Choose soft, slow music that mirrors the energy you want to invoke. Nothing jarring or sharp that may disturb the person from deep relaxation.

If you are someone who likes to adhere to a strict schedule when performing a session, you can search for timed music that makes a sound, like a gentle bell, every minute or every couple of minutes, letting you know to switch hand positions. Although, it is encouraged that you focus less on being exact with the timing and more on using intuition and the sensations you are feeling in your hands as a guide to switching positions.

You can certainly theme your selection to a chakra or element you are working with. For example, music with nature sounds for the Earth element or root chakra, rain sounds for the water element or sacral chakra, pianos or harps for the heart chakra, etc.

Several recommendations for Reiki music can be found in the resources section at the end of the book (see page 174).

SOUND HEALING

Sound healing is growing in popularity as an alternative healing modality. It encompasses the use of singing bowls (crystal or Tibetan), *Tingshas* (bells), chimes, tuning forks, gongs, and other instruments to restore vibrational harmony in the body. On its own, the music can be used to calm the nervous system, release blockages, and let go of emotions or thought patterns wreaking havoc in the mind and body.

It can be combined with Reiki in many different ways. But first, some of these instruments, such as gongs and singing bowls, can be quite expensive and difficult to transport (they are heavy and fragile!). Therefore, it is perfectly okay to research sound healing videos or search for sound healing playlists online to play as background music during a session—just download the playlist in advance and plug it into a decent speaker. If you do have access to these instruments or room in your budget (consider slowly acquiring different instruments), you can play them before, during, or after a session. You can also use the sound of the bells to let your clients know you are beginning a session or closing a session, and/or as a timer to let yourself know when you are switching positions.

Sound healing is wonderful for working with the throat chakra, the chakra that deals with balancing the vibrations and rhythms unique to our life. If you're working with singing bowls, different bowls produce different notes on the musical scale and correspond to each of the chakras. If you're in the market for a bowl, usually you'll see the notes labeled on the bottom of the bowl, or there will be a guide if you buy a seven-chakra set. As a rule of thumb, the larger the bowl, the deeper the vibration, which is associated with the lower chakras. Smaller bowls produce higher vibrations and can be used for the higher chakras.

TAPPING

Tapping, also known as the Emotional Freedom Technique, is another complementary energy healing tool, which works by targeting nine acupoints (meridians). It is used to rid feelings of pain, stress, anxiety, and depression. Like Reiki, it is noninvasive and painless, as you conduct the tapping with your hands and fingertips. However, anybody can do it—you don't need any special training or certification—so it can be great to combine both practices. So, how does it work? Before you begin the tapping, think about something unpleasant you may be currently going through, perhaps a feeling you need to release. Whatever it is, accept and acknowledge it. Say it verbally or in your head three times, and then begin the tapping sequence below. As you tap on each point, think of another statement to explain the reason behind your feelings, but say it just once.

- Start by making the palm of one hand flat, like a karate chop. With the pinky, ring, middle, and pointer fingertips of the other hand, tap into the fleshy side of the flat hand, between the wrist and the bottom of the pinky digit. Tap between five and seven times (and for each of the tapping points below, as well).

- Then move to the top of the eyebrow and tap.

- Move down below the eyebrow to the side of the face and tap at the bone near eye level.

- Now tap underneath the eye above the cheekbone.

- Tap underneath the nose.

- Tap between your bottom lip and your chin (in the crease).

Move to the collarbone—you may also use the whole hand to tap here.

Tap below your armpit.

Finally, tap the top of the head.

It doesn't matter which side of the body you conduct tapping on, as tapping works with the meridians, which are symmetrical. You may also choose to tap just one side of the body or do both at the same time using two hands where possible. The idea behind it is the acknowledgment of the feelings and doing so in a safe space. The tapping at these meridian points helps release the stuck energy and create new, positive thoughts to replace old, harmful thinking patterns. There is even evidence-based research to support the use of tapping for healing emotional distress.

Try tapping to work through common emotional issues tied to the lower chakras (see more in chapters 9 to 12). The very practice of love and acceptance of the self is great for the heart chakra in general. Below are some examples.

Root chakra: Even though I am not where I would like to be in my career, I love and accept myself.

Sacral chakra: Even though I feel upset, I love and accept myself.

Solar plexus chakra: Even though I am not as confident as I would like to be, I love and accept myself.

Heart chakra: Even though I struggle to let people into my life, I love and accept myself.

YOGA

Yoga, according to Patanjali (the father of modern yoga), is the cessation of the modifications or fluctuations of the mind. Yoga encompasses so many things, including the way we live, breathe, and meditate. In the West, the primary emphasis is typically on asana (postures), and asana is excellent to pair with a Reiki session. It not only promotes the circulation of prana (energy) in the body, but it can also be used to prepare for deep relaxation before a Reiki session. Practice these for anywhere from a couple of minutes to an hour before the Reiki session. Be sure to wind down the practice in corpse pose or meditation so you're ready to perform/receive Reiki. In fact, if you're a yoga teacher and a Reiki practitioner, during corpse pose is a wonderful time to provide a mini Reiki session. Hover or place your hands over the third eye chakra and/or cradle the back of the head with your palms. Below are some suggestions for asanas to target each chakra. You'll notice that many yogic asanas and sequences target multiple chakras at the same time.

Root: Lunges (crescent or high); warrior I, II, and III; tree pose; standing and full split; and child's pose. Focus on creating a solid foundation with the feet and the legs pressing firmly into the mat.

Sacral: Bound angle pose, lizard, goddess pose, warrior II, and extended side angle. Focus on postures that open either or both of the hips to the sides or tilt the hips forward and back (like cat-cow).

Solar Plexus: Boat pose, plank, twisting postures including twisted lunge, twisted chair pose, and seated spinal twist. The core should be emphasized during the practice by continuously drawing the navel in toward the spine.

Heart: Camel pose, bow pose, upward facing dog or baby cobra, wheel or bridge, flipped dog, and dancer's pose. Focus on drawing the shoulder blades closer together and broadening the collarbones to encourage opening in the chest and heart space.

Throat: Camel pose, shoulder stand or plow pose, fish pose to express the throat, or poses that involve drawing the throat toward the chin, such as pyramid pose or humble warrior.

Third Eye: Balancing postures such as eagle or tree, inversions such as headstand, handstand, or peacock. These are postures that involve a great deal of focus and mental strength.

Crown: Corpse pose, seated meditation, and pranayama (breathing). Allow yourself time and space to connect to your breath and the divinity within you.

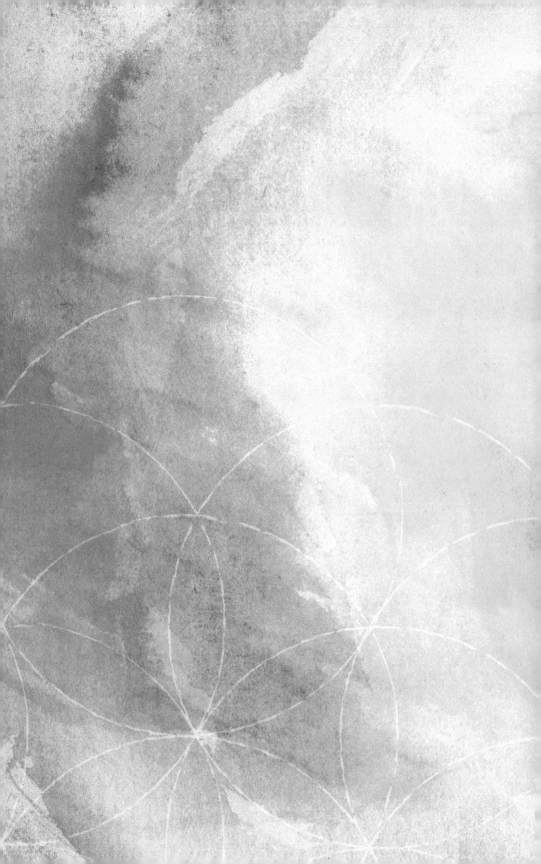

PART TWO

HEALING TECHNIQUES

Reiki is a great practice to bring balance to the chakras. In the same way, chakras are indicators of the possible emotional and spiritual reasons behind an ailment that can be relieved by a Reiki session. Both systems pair together beautifully.

Although Reiki will flow where it's needed, certain hand positions and symbols can help support specific chakras. Remember, everybody is different. Use these recommendations as starting points for your own exploration. Note the physical and emotional feelings that come up and notice how the same positions may feel different day after day. Some days you may feel a lot, others very little—that is entirely normal. Just keep going. The more you practice, the more sensitive you will become, and the more you will be able to let your intuition guide you.

CHAPTER 9

ROOT CHAKRA

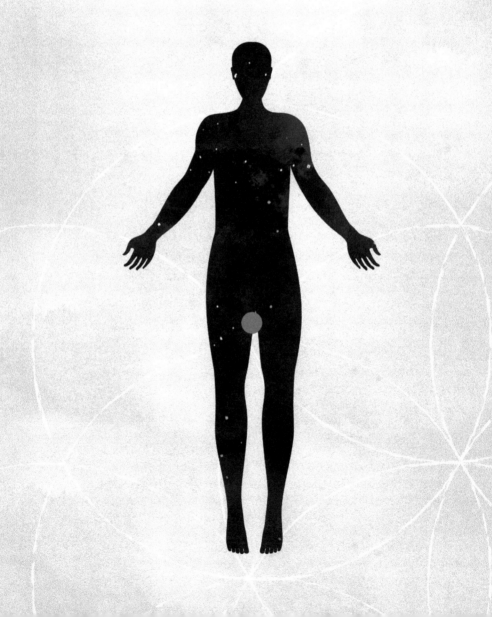

The first chakra is our spiritual foundation. To grow into strong and healthy beings, just like a tree, our roots need proper care and nourishment to support us. It's when one is over- or undernourished and supported that you can find imbalances here. Reiki healing, particularly with the hands-on approach, is a beautiful way to support the first chakra.

As a refresher, when thinking about the chakras, energy can go one of two ways. A deficiency is when too little energy is drawn into the chakra, and an excess is when too much energy is pouring into the chakra. These imbalances are what people refer to as blockages.

COMMON AILMENTS

THE PHYSICAL BODY

A balanced root chakra is reflective of someone who has overall good physical health. They have the tools, means, and/or self-care practices to support themselves. A strong root chakra is also linked with having a safe home environment, a stable source of income, and access to wholesome, nutritious food. All of the factors dealing with basic survival directly correlate to our physical health and this chakra.

It's when those factors are missing that there may be imbalances in the physical body. Of course, when someone doesn't eat well, is overly stressed about work or finances, or doesn't have sufficient health care, illnesses can develop. And sometimes, this stress is embedded even more deeply into our patterns and behaviors. For example, our eating habits are affected by the root chakra. A deficient chakra may result in someone who is malnourished, while an excessive chakra may result in someone who overeats or carries too much weight in their body in an effort to find grounding. Another potential pattern is feeling sluggish and weighed down by the pressures of surviving in this world. Because the root chakra is related to stability and sits at the lowest point of our spine, our lower extremities (feet and legs), bones, low back, and immune system may be impacted by imbalances. The body parts directly responsible for holding us up and keeping us together become compromised.

THE EMOTIONAL, MENTAL, AND SPIRITUAL BODY

Tuning in to the power of the root chakra is the definition of grounding, literally. Balance and relief are achieved when we feel stable and calm and trust that we have the means to handle whatever circumstances come our way. We are unable to be stirred, trusting in the Earth's protection. A balanced root chakra also enables us to be in the present moment. Feeling grateful and trusting that where we are now is exactly where we need to be.

When that trust is not there, there may be emotional, mental, and spiritual imbalances. Anxiety, fear, and dread can come in and affect our confidence, our energy, and even our will to carry on. Because the root chakra carries with it ancestral and womb memories, imbalances can also result if there are unhealed generational traumas or issues with family. Someone with a weak root chakra feels either ungrounded or dissociated. This can also happen if too much energy is focused on the higher chakras—an inability to come back down to Earth, so to speak, or to prioritize basic needs. To take things in the other direction, if too much energy is centered in the root chakra, you might find someone who is overly cocky, obsessing over material things and unable to connect to spirit. Remembering the upward directional flow of prana, if energy is stuck in the first chakra, it can't move up to support the functions of the higher chakras. So, as it has been described earlier, the first chakra is really our spiritual foundation! It is key to maturing as a healthy and productive human being.

HAND POSITIONS

This is a great sequence to support your root chakra. It focuses on the area where it's located and its area of influence. The last position is a great way to bring balance by connecting the earthy quality of this chakra to the most heavenly one (crown).

1. Take three deep breaths into your hara to center yourself.

2. Place your hands in Gassho to set your intention to receive the healing needed and bring balance to that energy center. You can come up with your own wording, but try to keep it as open as possible—sometimes, the imbalance in one chakra is related to another one, and you don't want to limit the impact of the session.

3. Place your hands on your groin for two to three minutes. Keep your awareness on your hands and groin.

4. Move your hands to the abdomen. Keep them there for two to three minutes. Again, place your awareness on that area of your body.

5. Move them to the lower back. Keep your hands there for two to three minutes, focusing your awareness there.

6. Place your hands on your knees for two to three minutes.

7. Place one hand on your groin, the other one on the crown. Let the energy flow between your hands. You can visualize a white light going from the top of your head to the groin at the inhale, and from the groin to the top of your head on the exhale.

8. End the sequence by placing your hands in Gassho to give thanks for the healing received.

TIP FOR SESSIONS WITH OTHERS. This protocol (and all the chakra protocols included in this book) can also be used on a recipient. You may want to let your hands hover over positions like the groin instead of touching them directly.

SYMBOLS AND MANTRAS

To promote balance in the root chakra, working with the Power symbol, CKR, is ideal. CKR is linked to the earth energy—our connection to life, grounding, sense of safety and stability—which is the perfect environment for this center to thrive.

You can work with CKR to bring balance to your root chakra in many ways:

Option 1:

1. Draw CKR in the air or in front of your root chakra, repeat its mantra three times to activate it, and then bring the symbol into your root chakra (groin) using your hands.

2. Keep this hand position for five minutes, placing all of your awareness in your hands.

3. Some Reiki lineages draw CKR directly on the palms of the hands and then place these on the chakra.

4. Close with Gassho to give thanks.

   Note: Remember to draw the symbol slowly and with awareness.

Option 2:

1. Visualize CKR inside the area of your body associated with your root chakra (groin/base of the spine).

2. Activate it by chanting its mantra three times.

3. Breathe in and out normally, keeping your awareness on the symbol and the base of your spine. If you don't have a steady meditation practice, do it for only a few breaths. If you do, try to do this visualization from 10 to 15 minutes. Keeping your hands in the groin position during this meditation will help you stay focused on that area.

4. Close with Gassho to give thanks.

Option 3:

1. Chant the mantra Choku Rei for five to 10 minutes.

2. Chant from your hara to make your root chakra vibrate with the energy of the earth.

3. Close with Gassho to give thanks.

TIP FOR SESSIONS WITH OTHERS. Chant silently or visualize CKR while letting your hands hover on the root chakra.

CHAPTER 10

SACRAL CHAKRA

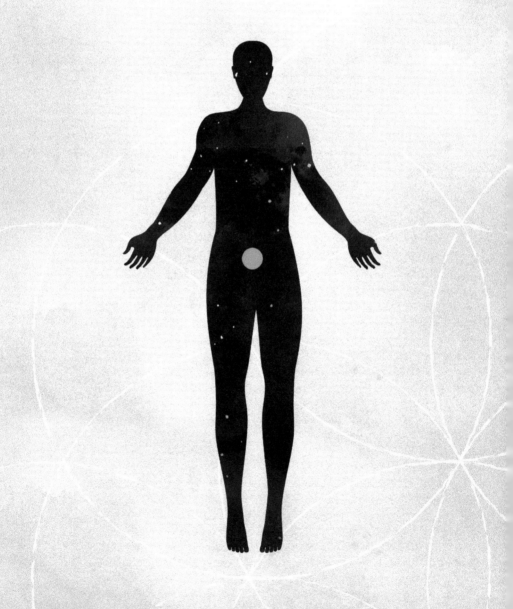

The water-like characteristics of the sacral chakra, including sexuality, fluidity, and emotions, are key to our health and vitality. Humans need the freedom to explore themselves and the world around them—to find hobbies, activities, and people who bring us pleasure. It is also necessary to recognize our right to feel but not allow our feelings to overcome us. The practice of Reiki in and of itself is supportive of freeing blockages and restoring the fluid movement of ki in the body. It can also greatly help with emotional regulation by encouraging the release of harmful thought patterns and feelings that don't serve us. Reiki encourages self-exploration and strengthens the mind-body connection.

~~~~~~~~

COMMON AILMENTS

THE PHYSICAL BODY

The sexual and reproductive organs, impacting our ability to procreate, are the core of the sacral chakra. A balanced chakra enables sexual pleasure. It also includes our reproductive capability and healthy menstruation for women. Since the sacral chakra includes our pelvis and hips, it is also linked to mobility and movement. While most of the digestive system sits in the solar plexus chakra, the large intestine is in the sacral chakra. It and our urinary tract system deal with the healthy elimination of water and waste from the body.

Sexual and reproductive health is affected by an imbalanced sacral chakra. One might find deficiencies show up in the physical body, such as an inability to feel pleasure during sex, impotency, or issues with menstruation for women. Yoga teachers commonly say that our emotions live in our hips as they guide us through hip-opening poses. And what happens when there is not much movement or we close ourselves off? It can exacerbate sadness and depression, cause mobility issues in the hips, and limit flexibility. Lastly, emotional blockages in the sacral chakra can result in lower back pain and tension and can inhibit prana from moving up the spine to our higher chakras.

THE EMOTIONAL, MENTAL, AND SPIRITUAL BODY

Our emotions are directly tied to the sacral chakra! Balance is reflective of someone who is in control of their emotions. It's about letting the emotions flow in (allowing yourself to feel) but also letting the emotions go as appropriate, similar to the elimination function in the physical body. A balanced sacral chakra also includes having an open mind and allowing yourself to take pleasure in the things that make you happy. Exploration, adventure, and creation are all important to the emotional, mental, and spiritual health of the sacral chakra.

If one is imbalanced or deficient in the sacral chakra, they may be emotionally and spiritually cold, feeling numb and not open to or interested in trying new things. It can also show up as someone who is unable to feel pleasure, either sexual pleasure or even pleasure from regular or seemingly "fun" activities. And if there is pleasure, there may be guilt attached to it—a feeling of "I don't deserve to be enjoying myself right now." When there is too much energy flowing into the chakra, there can be too-intense emotions, and not in a good way. Hello, drama! You might find someone who is very sensitive, susceptible to mood swings, and unable to handle their emotions if things fall out of their control.

HAND POSITIONS

These specific hand positions help support a proper balance in your sacral chakra. As with the root chakra, we are giving the final balancing touch by connecting this second chakra to the second to last chakra (third eye). Remember: Don't try too hard—just enjoy your practice and let the energy flow. *Enjoyment* is a keyword for the sacral chakra.

1. Take three deep breaths into your hara to center yourself.

2. Place your hands in Gassho to set your intention to receive the healing needed and bring balance to the sacral chakra.

3. Place your hands on your abdomen for two to three minutes. Keep your awareness on your

hands and abdomen (center your focus on a point closer to the spine than the skin).

4. Move your hands to the lower back. Keep them there for two to three minutes. Again, place your awareness on that area of your body.

5. Move them to the groin. Keep your hands there for two to three minutes, focusing your awareness there.

6. Place one hand on your abdomen, the other one on the forehead. Let the energy flow between your hands. You can visualize a white light going from the forehead to the abdomen on the inhale, and from the abdomen to the forehead on the exhale.

7. End the sequence by placing your hands in Gassho to give thanks for the healing received.

TIP FOR SESSIONS WITH OTHERS. You can do this protocol in the same order with the recipient seated on a chair. If the person is lying down, do the front positions first. Then ask the person to lie on their stomach and do the lower back. Remember to hover in sensitive places!

SYMBOLS AND MANTRAS

The Power symbol, CKR, brings qualities like confidence, vitality, and clarity to the sacral chakra. However, the water element and fluid quality of this chakra are also related to the heavenly energy of the Harmony symbol, SHK.

Here are two ways to combine CKR and SHK to bring balance to your sacral chakra:

Option 1:

1. Draw CKR in the air or in front of your sacral chakra, repeat its mantra three times to activate it, and bring the symbol into your sacral chakra (abdomen) using your hands. Some Reiki lineages draw CKR directly on the palms of the hands and then place these on the chakra.

2. Keep this hand position for five minutes, putting all of your awareness in your hands.

3. Let go of this position, breathe normally a few times, and then repeat the same process with SHK, but for only two to three minutes.

4. Close with Gassho to give thanks.

Option 2:

1. Visualize CKR inside the area of your body associated with your sacral chakra (abdomen). Activate it by repeating its mantra three times.

2. Breathe in and out normally for five to 10 minutes, keeping your awareness on the symbol and your abdomen.

3. Let go of the CKR symbol. Take a few deep breaths and visualize SKH, the Harmony symbol, within your whole body for three to five minutes.

4. Let go of the symbol; close with Gassho to give thanks.

TIP FOR SESSIONS WITH OTHERS. Chant silently or visualize the first CKR, then SHK, while letting your hands hover or lightly touch that chakra.

CHAPTER 11

SOLAR PLEXUS CHAKRA

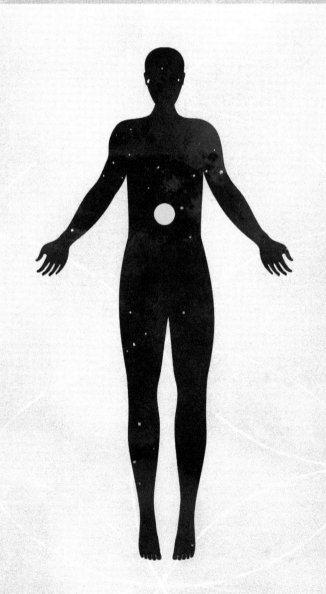

Our solar plexus chakra, situated within our core, enables us to carry out actions to our heart's content. Described as our energy center, when brightly lit, it helps give us the confidence and willpower to thrive. Reiki practice can help energize this chakra and bring light and warmth where it is needed. It can also calm the sympathetic nervous system, which is often responsible for causing excess fear and anxiety.

COMMON AILMENTS

THE PHYSICAL BODY

The solar plexus chakra includes our abdomen and the organs of our digestive tract, such as the small intestine, stomach, pancreas, gallbladder, and liver. It also includes our adrenal glands, which are responsible for the production of cortisol (helps regulate metabolism and response to stress). Lastly, it includes our muscular system. Physical balance in this chakra includes healthy digestion, nutrient absorption, and energy levels, along with good muscle mass.

Food is broken down (transformed) in the small intestine to give us nutrients and energy to perform the activities of our daily lives. Thus, imbalances in the solar plexus chakra can affect this process, causing a range of digestive disorders and lethargy. Even if eating a lot of nutritious foods, someone experiencing a deficiency in this chakra can still end up constantly feeling tired and the need to supplement their diet with stimulants like coffee or amphetamines. A deficient solar plexus could also result in someone who carries a lot of weight around their internal organs, which can cause chronic diseases like obesity and diabetes. Someone who is physically weak (has no muscle mass) may also experience a deficiency. However, an excess imbalance can show up as someone who metabolizes food too quickly or hypoglycemia.

THE EMOTIONAL, MENTAL, AND SPIRITUAL BODY

The solar plexus chakra is responsible for providing us with confidence, willpower, and motivation. It impacts our reactions to all those things that give us butterflies in our stomach—like taking risks, standing up for ourselves, or speaking in front of a large audience. Characteristics of a balanced chakra include the ability to be confident, courageous, and self-disciplined—qualities that are necessary to enable us to take action or make changes. Our solar plexus chakra also includes our ego and our identity, so someone with a balanced chakra has a good sense of their identity and good self-esteem. Metaphorically, the balance of this chakra is a flame—heat and warmth are necessary to ignite the inner fire within us, but not to the point of an uncontrollable blaze.

Both emerging science and traditional Eastern medicine posit that the health of our gut and other organs, such as the liver, impacts our emotions. Therefore, an imbalance in the solar plexus chakra could result in anxiety or anger (excess), or fear or depression (deficiency). Because this chakra deals with our ego and identity, a deficiency can show up as someone who has low self-esteem. It may also be someone who fears taking risks or making changes for fear of their own bright light shining. On the flip side, an excessive chakra can exhibit in being overly aggressive, cocky, and controlling. Perhaps it is someone who takes risks only for the ego boost or the rush (an adrenaline junkie), rather than as part of a personal mission. You also might find someone who lives with constant anxiety, even when there is no real danger.

HAND POSITIONS

The solar plexus chakra is also the center for transformation. Keep this word in mind while doing hands-on healing. Pay special attention to even the smallest change you feel in your body, energy, thoughts, or feelings. Don't engage, don't judge, just observe them—a still mind amid a sea of change.

1. Take three deep breaths into your hara to center yourself.

2. Place your hands in Gassho to set your intention to receive the healing needed and bring balance to the solar plexus chakra.

3. Place your hands on your middle back for two to three minutes. Keep your awareness on your hands and middle back (center your focus on a point closer to the spine than the skin).

4. Move your hands to the lower back. Keep them there for two to three minutes. Again, place your awareness on that area of your body.

5. Move them to your navel. Keep your hands there for two to three minutes, focusing your awareness there.

6. Place one hand on your navel, the other one on the heart. Let the energy flow between your hands. This placement is known as the universal balancing position. It's a great go-to placement when you have no time and need a quick Reiki pick-me-up.

7. End the sequence by placing your hands in Gassho to give thanks for the healing received.

TIP FOR SESSIONS WITH OTHERS. If your recipient is a female, let your hands hover during the universal balancing position. You can also place the tips of the index and middle fingers on the heart area above the breasts.

SYMBOLS AND MANTRAS

The solar plexus is related to the adrenal and digestive systems, in terms of physicality. These are tied to the capacity to let fear go and see reality as it is. In this way, we can take the right action and set healthy self-boundaries. All of these are qualities boosted by the Power symbol, CKR, and its focusing and grounding energy.

Working with CKR to balance your solar plexus:

1. Draw CKR in front of you. Activate it by repeating its mantra three times.

2. Slowly bring the CKR symbol inside your body. Visualize it there for three to five minutes, and then let go of the symbol.

3. Take a few deep breaths and visualize CKR in your solar plexus (navel). Place your hands on this chakra and focus your awareness there for three minutes.

4. Place your hands on your middle back for three minutes, visualizing the symbol inside your solar plexus.

5. Let go of the symbol and stay in the energetic space you created for a minute or two.

6. Close with Gassho to give thanks.

TIP FOR SESSIONS WITH OTHERS. If your recipient is sitting on a chair, you can place your hands on the shoulders while you visualize CKR inside the whole body. If the person is lying down, you can put one hand on the solar plexus and the other one just above the heart area.

CHAPTER 12

HEART CHAKRA

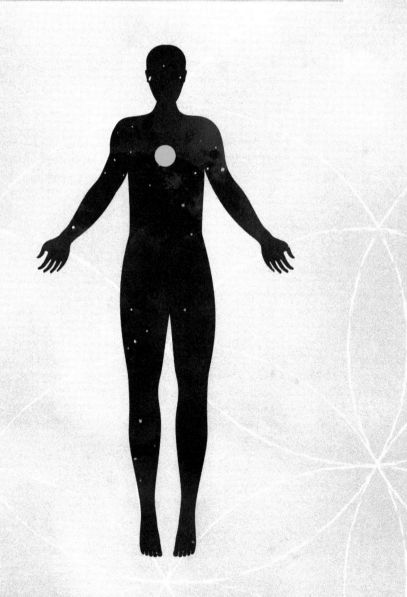

The heart chakra, as its Sanskrit name says, is "unhurt," and so should be the flow of energy as it traverses through this chakra—the midpoint between the lower, more material chakras to the higher, more spiritual chakras. It deals with our love of self and others. Reiki practice promotes kindness and acceptance, which are healing to the heart chakra. It also encourages us to let go and release traumas we might be holding on to subconsciously.

COMMON AILMENTS

THE PHYSICAL BODY

The organs of the heart chakra include, of course, the heart and circulatory system, lungs, and other organs responsible for respiration. This chakra also includes the shoulders, arms, and hands. The heart chakra is essential for keeping our whole system functioning and delivering precious oxygen and blood to our entire body. In the heart chakra, balance looks like optimal, unrestricted breathing and circulation.

When there is an imbalance in the heart chakra, air or blood flow can be blocked or restricted. There might be issues in the respiratory tract or problems with respiration or the circulatory system—for example, shortness of breath, asthma, heart attack, or stroke. Similar to the hips—the ball and socket joint explored in the sacral chakra—our shoulders and chest (and arms and hands) are also used to convey how we want to interact with others. For example, people who experience a deficiency in their heart chakra may turn themselves inward (visible in a notorious crunched back and rounded shoulders), or avoid embracing others. When the chest is compressed, there is trouble breathing. An excess may be someone whose chest protrudes too far, someone who wears their heart on their sleeve, so to speak, or someone who gives too much of themselves away. Breathing too far into the chest is not good for respiration either, as we don't end up taking full, quality breaths to nourish ourselves. Either stance can restrict the flow of prana to the other chakras.

Love (of self and others), kindness, compassion, trust, peace, and harmony are all associated with a balanced heart chakra. There is also a delicate balance of giving and receiving. Healers and/or other nurturers, in particular, tend to expend a lot of energy on helping others, so it is particularly important for them not to neglect self-care to feel balanced. The heart chakra also deals with living in the present moment, rather than allowing past circumstances or future worries dictate our joy.

Everyone wants to be loved and accepted by themselves and others. It is devastating to the heart chakra to lose a loved one and have the heart broken (or vice versa), and to live a life without love. Deficiencies in this chakra can cause someone to turn themselves inward and close themselves off to others. It may also inhibit one's ability to be compassionate and empathetic toward others. How many times does it happen that when someone is hurting, they tend to hurt someone else—either intentionally or unintentionally? Thus, relationships can suffer on many levels. If there is an excess in the heart chakra, you will find someone who may give too much—a martyr type or someone who is not able to set healthy boundaries. It is also common to see someone who may cling to people and past relationships, when what they really need is to let go. These emotional circumstances, either holding on too tightly or letting go of too much, cause disruptions to the flow of energy in the physical body.

HAND POSITIONS

To open your heart and bring balance to this center, you need to feel safe. This means that beyond the obvious positions in the torso—where the heart chakra is located—and shoulders, it's essential to give some love to the root chakra as well. Take time to explore what feels good for you.

1. Take three deep breaths into your hara to center yourself.

2. Place your hands in Gassho to set your intention to receive the healing needed and bring balance to the heart chakra.

3. Place your hands on your groin for two to three minutes. Keep your awareness on your hands and groin (center your focus on a point close to the spine).

4. Move your hands to your heart. Keep them there for two to three minutes. Again, place your awareness on that area of your body.

5. Move your hands to your shoulders. Keep them there for two to three minutes. Feel the warmth of your hands melting the tension away and your shoulders moving away from your ears.

6. Place your hands in the middle back and let the energy flow for two to three minutes.

7. End by placing your hands in Gassho to give thanks for the healing received.

TIP FOR SESSIONS WITH OTHERS. When treating others, starting with the groin can feel a bit invasive. You may want to switch the order and start with the shoulders, then follow with heart and groin. Then turn the recipient to lie on their stomach and treat the back.

SYMBOLS AND MANTRAS

The heart chakra and the third Reiki symbol, HSZSN, are a match made in heaven. They both share the same qualities of unconditional love and compassion. Working with HSZSN will open your heart center and strengthen it. By doing so, you will feel more compassionate toward others and have a stronger connection during sessions. Additionally, you will feel more compassionate toward yourself and bring much-needed forgiveness and love into your life.

However, to be able to open your heart, it is always a good idea to support this chakra with some grounding energy, which means adding a touch of the Power symbol.

Open your heart using CKR and HSZSN:

1. Visualize CKR inside your whole body.

2. Activate it by repeating its mantra three times.

3. Breathe in and out normally, visualizing CKR for five to ten minutes.

4. Let go of the symbol. Stay in the energetic space you created for a minute or two.

5. Take a few deep breaths, and then visualize HSZSN in your heart area for five to ten minutes. Try to feel the energy of the symbol inside your heart (not in front), if possible. You can place your hands on your heart or in Gassho to help keep your mind focused on this area.

6. Let go of the symbol.

7. Stay in the energetic space you created for a minute or two.

8. Close with Gassho to give thanks.

TIP FOR SESSIONS WITH OTHERS. Chant silently, or visualize first, CKR and then SHSK, while placing your hands on the heart chakra. You can visualize the symbol inside the recipient's body or in the space between both of you.

CHAPTER 13

THROAT
CHAKRA

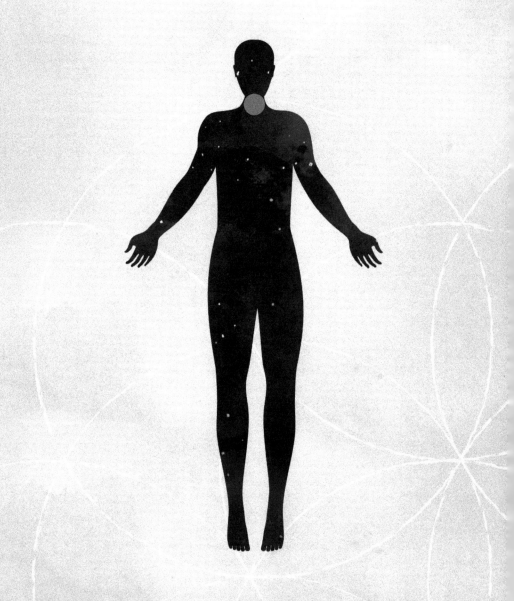

The throat chakra is responsible for verbal and non-verbal communication and our ability to listen. It also deals with self-expression, sharing our truth, and conveying needs and desires. Therefore, it is key to feeling whole. Reiki practice allows us to tune in to our bodies. When there is space for quiet reflection, it is possible to better understand what our bodies need to heal and also how to live an authentic life.

~~~~~~~~

COMMON AILMENTS

THE PHYSICAL BODY

Another chakra whose name speaks for itself, the throat chakra, includes our throat, ears, mouth (teeth, tongue, and gums), thyroid, hypothalamus, and speech organs. Its Sanskrit name *Vishuddha*, which translates to "purification," means it also deals with toxicities in the body. With a balanced throat chakra, one would have good oral health and no issues with speech or hearing. The body would also be free of toxicities.

Imbalances in the throat chakra may include speech or hearing impairments or problems with the jaw. Imbalances can also include toxicities in the body, which could have a larger effect on all of our systems. The thyroid, responsible for the production of hormones that deal with metabolism and regulating body temperature can suffer if there is an imbalance in the throat chakra. It is common in healing spaces, and in general, for the throat area to be one of the most sensitive regions of the body to work with. Why? Because speaking up or speaking our truth in any setting can make us feel extremely vulnerable. Hence, the lump in the throat that is experienced during uncomfortable situations. Sometimes this results in tension in the neck and jaw.

THE EMOTIONAL, MENTAL, AND SPIRITUAL BODY

The throat chakra is the first chakra that starts to reach into the spiritual realm, dealing with the vibrations perceived (from listening) and the ones put forth (by speaking). In the physical sense, it's also the passageway between our heart and mind. The challenge is how to communicate from both places and not let energy get trapped in between the two places. As such, this chakra is often referred to as a "bottleneck" for energy. Balance in the throat chakra looks like someone who is able to safely express themself. What's pure is also what's truthful, so an important aspect for the health of the throat chakra is to able to share your truth and to be awake to others' truths by being a good listener.

The throat chakra can become unbalanced if it doesn't feel safe to express ourselves and may exhibit deficiencies, such as trouble communicating, difficulty being able to share what's on our mind, or issues with consenting to something. This is why it's important to achieve good health in the lower chakras, as they will give us the foundation for being able to vocalize our needs and desires. Other characteristics of an unbalanced chakra in a deficiency also include being overly quiet or shy and unable to share creative thoughts and ideas. Excesses may show up as someone who talks too much without doing enough listening. It may also be someone who is too loud, overshadowing others. When it comes to purification, this also includes the energy that is put out into this world. This chakra in excess may look like someone who, when they talk, is either negative or cynical, or talks behind others' backs.

HAND POSITIONS

The area of the throat chakra is very sensitive when it comes to hands-on healing. Go slowly and monitor your feelings. If it becomes too intense, hover your hands instead of using touch. In this protocol, we will also support the chakras above (clear vision) and below (feelings) the throat chakra.

1. Take three deep breaths into your hara to center yourself.

2. Place your hands in Gassho to set your intention to receive the healing needed and bring balance to the throat chakra.

3. Place your hands in front of both eyes for two to three minutes. Feel the warmth of your hands relaxing every muscle of your eyes and surrounding area.

4. Move your hands to your ears, with the heels of your hands resting on the jaw. Stay there for two to three minutes.

5. Move your hands to your throat. Keep them there for three to five minutes. You can intensify this process by asking questions and noticing any change in energy. For example, "What am I not saying that needs to be said?" "What stops me from expressing my truth?" "What scares me from sharing my feelings?"

6. Move your hands to your heart for two to three minutes.

7. Place your hands on the groin, and let the energy flow for one to two minutes for grounding and

building a sense of safety that will allow you to speak your truth.

8. End with Gassho to give thanks for the healing received.

TIP FOR SESSIONS WITH OTHERS. Always avoid touching the throat of a recipient, unless asked to do so. You can do this sequence twice, once on the front of the body and once on the back.

SYMBOLS AND MANTRAS

The throat chakra's essence of "speaking your truth" resonates strongly with the Master symbol, DKM, which represents your bright inner light and true essence. Remember, when working with DKM, balance it with grounding modalities to avoid becoming too spacey. If you are a Reiki 2 practitioner and have not worked with DKM yet, check out the variation included at the end of this chapter.

Working with DKM for the throat chakra:

1. Set your hands in Gassho and set the intention to reconnect with your true self.

2. Visualize a bright sphere of light over your head with DKM in the center.

3. Visualize this bright sphere of light entering your crown and going down your head until it's located in your throat. Let it stay there for one to two minutes.

4. Visualize the bright sphere of light going down your spine and all the way down into the Earth, clearing your whole central channel.

5. Repeat two more times, for a total of three passes.

6. Stay in the energetic space you have created for a minute or two.

7. Close with Gassho to give thanks.

VARIATION FOR REIKI 2 PRACTITIONERS. Perform one pass with CKR, one pass with SHK, and one with HSZSN.

TIP FOR SESSIONS WITH OTHERS. Adapt this technique by letting your hands hover over the recipient's crown and then moving them slowly from crown to throat. Hover over the throat for one to two minutes, and then gently move your hands over the rest of the body, sweeping the energy to the earth after going over the feet.

CHAPTER 14

THIRD EYE CHAKRA

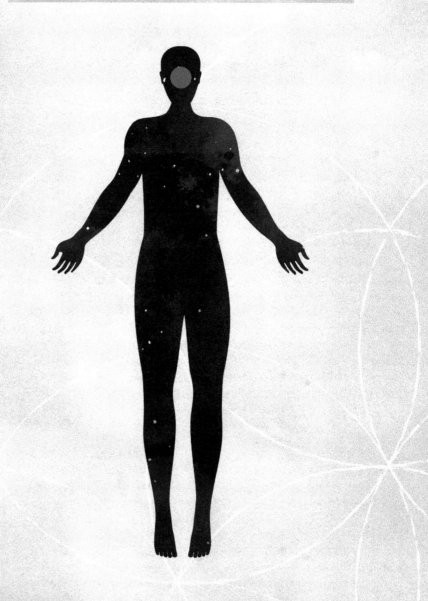

As for the third eye chakra, ailments deal more with matters of the mind. The third eye chakra is associated with light, and its main qualities include illumination, intuition, and clarity. Many people who practice and receive Reiki do so for its mental benefits. Reiki can help remove the cloudiness and fog that build up in the mirror of ourselves and within our minds over a lifetime.

~~~~~~~~

COMMON AILMENTS

THE PHYSICAL BODY

The third eye chakra sits in our head behind our brows, and it includes our eyes, our nose, parts of our brain, and our neurological system. Therefore, balance in this chakra in the physical sense includes good neurological health and good vision. The pineal gland is also located in the region of this chakra and is responsible for the production of melatonin. So, this chakra also deals with the balance of our circadian rhythm—producing a healthy sleep-wake cycle. Our circadian rhythm is affected by exposure to light and darkness, so it makes sense that our environment and lifestyle (the hours we work, our exposure to sunlight, etc.) can affect the balance of our internal clock.

In the third eye chakra, physical imbalances may include experiencing frequent headaches, migraines, and/or poor vision. Neurological issues include seizures and other disorders. One's psychological health may also suffer in a number of ways (e.g., anxiety, depression). An imbalance in the sixth chakra can also impact sleep. For example, one may experience trouble sleeping, trouble remembering dreams (deficiency), or frequent nightmares (excess). Lastly, there can be problems with sinuses.

THE EMOTIONAL, MENTAL, AND SPIRITUAL BODY

Particularly within the spiritual community, many people strive to achieve balance in the third eye chakra. Wisdom, intuition, perception, open-mindedness, and imagination to think big to actualize our wildest dreams, and help others do the same, are all parts of the third eye chakra. In addition to these qualities, having a balanced third eye chakra also includes the ability to remain focused, the ability to visualize, and a good memory. It's also a fine balance of perceiving what is real (true or possible) and what is not. In order to achieve this state of balance, there must be groundedness and compassion to overcome the fears and anxieties that get in the way of staying focused and connecting to our true selves.

When the third eye chakra is unbalanced, it affects our ability to see clearly. There may be confusion about who we are and what path we should be on. It can also affect our interpretation of things (even ourselves)—the range of being spot on or way off to what is true. Unfortunately, a lack of balance can lead to a lack of understanding of our life's purpose, and even if we do understand it, we may not have the tools to manifest whatever it may be. This lack of clarity can be experienced from the side of a deficiency or an excess. For example, a deficient third eye chakra can include poor imagination, inability to visualize, and closed-mindedness—for example, someone who doesn't or cannot believe in anything. If there is an excess, you might find someone who is delusional, a daydreamer who is unable to focus or is out of touch with reality.

HAND POSITIONS

To support the third eye chakra, use positions that bring clarity of vision. The first position in this sequence, for example, is helpful to let go of patterns that no longer work for you, and embrace new perspectives. (You can do it on its own for a few minutes when you feel stuck.) In the same way we used this chakra to balance the sacral, now we are using the sacral chakra to give the final balancing touch to the third eye.

1. Take three deep breaths into your hara to center yourself.

2. Place your hands in Gassho to set your intention to receive the healing needed and bring balance to the third eye chakra.

3. Place one hand on the back of the head, and the other on the forehead. Let the energy flow between both hands for two to three minutes.

4. Move your hands to your throat. Keep them there for two to three minutes.

5. Move your hands to the eyes. Stay there for three to five minutes. Feel the energy flowing inside your head, softening and relaxing.

6. Place one hand on the forehead and one on the sacral chakra area (abdomen) for balancing. Do this for two to three minutes.

7. End by placing your hands in Gassho to give thanks for the healing received.

TIP FOR SESSIONS WITH OTHERS. If the recipient is not allergic to or distracted by scent, you can use soothing lavender or chamomile scented oils or balms on your hands while you do the eye position.

SYMBOLS AND MANTRAS

The third eye chakra area is the perfect home for the Harmony symbol, SHK, which will strengthen the connection to the spirit, promote intuition, and give clarity of vision. To bring it into your daily life and avoid becoming too spacey, however, it's ideal to anchor this heavenly energy with the grounding quality of the Power symbol, CKR.

1. Visualize SHK inside the area associated with the third eye (forehead). Try to place your awareness inside your head instead of outside.

2. Activate it by repeating its mantra three times.

3. Breathe in and out normally, keeping your awareness on the symbol and your forehead for five minutes.

4. Pay attention to any feelings, thoughts, or sensations that take place.

5. Let go of SHK, and stay for a minute or two in the energetic space you created.

6. Visualize CKR inside your body.

7. Activate it by repeating its mantra three times.

8. Keep visualizing CKR for five to ten minutes.

9. Let go of CKR, and stay for a minute or two in the energetic space you created.

10. Close with Gassho to give thanks.

TIP FOR SESSIONS WITH OTHERS. Start with your hands placed lightly on the recipient's eyes while visualizing or chanting SHK silently. Then place one hand on the crown and the other one on the abdomen while visualizing or chanting CKR silently.

CHAPTER 15

CROWN CHAKRA

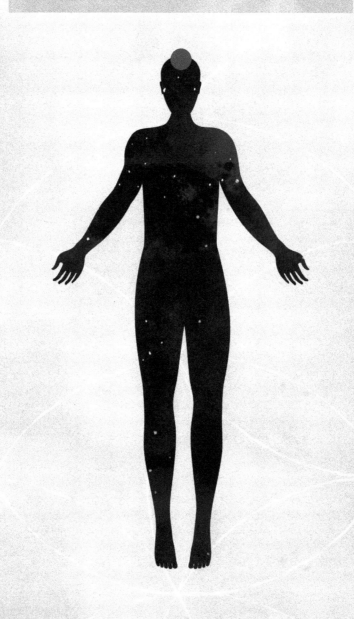

The last chakra is the crown chakra, the point of transcendence. Accessing the crown chakra allows us to leave our bodies and connect to spirit (whatever that may mean on an individual level), experiencing true bliss. It also gives us a sense of interconnectedness to the universe—allowing us to feel "at one." Through a consistent Reiki practice, we can connect with heavenly energy and feel guided by a higher power. This, in and of itself, can be extremely healing.

COMMON AILMENTS

THE PHYSICAL BODY

Where or what is the "crown" exactly? Quite literally it's the place where a queen or king's crown would fall, at the very top of the head. Physically, the crown chakra deals with consciousness and cognitive functioning. A balanced crown chakra includes having a healthy brain and a sound mind. While there is some debate, the pituitary gland also sits in the crown chakra. Its function, along with maintaining our body chemistry, is to regulate the hormone glands below it (both physically and those that reside in the lower chakras). Therefore, the pituitary is also known as the "master gland."

Physical imbalances (disturbances) to the crown chakra are among some of the most devastating, including cancer, amnesia, brain tumors, comas, and psychosis. However, some may also experience imbalances in a less serious matter, such as feeling dizzy or dissociated. Headaches and migraines can also be experienced here. Lastly, one may experience hormonal imbalances or conditions of the pituitary gland.

THE EMOTIONAL, MENTAL, AND SPIRITUAL BODY

To access the crown chakra, let alone achieve balance, is an ongoing, lifelong practice. The crown chakra can be thought of as a master to all the other chakras because there must first be balance in the lower chakras to have made it to this point. Qualities of this chakra include "feeling at one," interconnectedness to the universe and other beings, and liberation from worldly matters, leading to bliss. While this spiritual stuff all sounds nice, on a daily basis, what it really means for balance is our ability to be mindful and thoughtful human beings. In other words, we are able to view things from a universal perspective so there is no separateness from one another. It is also having faith in a higher power.

It is not a quick or easy process to access the crown chakra. Therefore, do not get down on yourself or others if you or they are not quite there yet. However, imbalances to look for (or spaces to work on) with this chakra deal with consciousness and spirituality. A deficient crown chakra can be reflected by an inability to connect to spirit or someone who is too narrow-minded in their belief systems. It can also include someone who is stuck in the lower chakras—focused too heavily on material attachments (perhaps fame or fortune) to have an awareness of existence beyond this Earth. It can also show up as feeling lonely or disconnected and a lack of interest in life. In excess, a crown chakra imbalance is experienced as someone who may be too spacey or too stuck up in the clouds and who needs to come back down to Earth, common for healers or energy workers. This is why it is so important to balance heavenly energy with grounding. We can use heavenly energy for guidance and healing, but on a daily basis, it is important to live in this world and be on the same level as everyone else to function.

HAND POSITIONS

For the crown chakra to open, all the others have to bloom first. This sequence is inspired by that principle, bringing balance from the root chakra up—an energetic journey that takes you from Earth to heaven.

1. Take three deep breaths into your hara to center yourself.

2. Place your hands in Gassho to set your intention to receive the healing needed and bring balance to the crown chakra.

3. Place your hands on the groin (root) for one to two minutes. Let the energy flow.

4. Move your hands to the abdomen (sacral) for one to two minutes.

5. Move your hands to your navel (solar plexus) for one to two minutes.

6. Move your hands to the heart for one to two minutes.

7. Move your hands to your throat for one to two minutes.

8. Move your hands to your forehead for one to two minutes.

9. Move your hands to the top of your head for one to two minutes.

10. Keep one hand on the top of your head and move the other one to the groin for a minute or two for the final balancing touch.

11. End with Gassho to give thanks for the healing received.

TIP FOR SESSIONS WITH OTHERS. Do this on both the front and the back. Remember to hover on sensitive areas! Playlists that use natural elements can be an excellent enhancement to this session. (Check the resources section on page 174 for suggestions.)

SYMBOLS AND MANTRAS

The crown chakra is all about the connection with the source, which is embodied in its maximum expression by DKM. When we step into DKM energy, we feel a shower of luminous energy filling our whole body. Through the following meditation, we bring that energy from the crown to the root to help balance our entire energetic system.

Working with DKM for the crown chakra:

1. Set your hands in Gassho and set the intention to reconnect with your true self.

2. Raise your arms perpendicular to your head, palms facing each other.

3. Feel the energy flowing between your hands.

4. Visualize DKM in that space. Activate it by repeating its mantra three times. When you feel the connection with the symbol, turn the palms to face your crown. Imagine the energy falling like a waterfall on your body from the crown down.

5. Do this for a minute or so. Then move your hands down, three to four inches away from the front of your body. Your palms are facing in. It's almost like you are sweeping the energy down the front of your body and into the earth. Do this slowly and with awareness.

6. Repeat this two more times for a total of three passes.

7. Stay in the energetic space you created for a minute or two.

8. Close with Gassho to give thanks.

VARIATION FOR REIKI 2 PRACTITIONERS. Perform one pass with CKR, one pass with SHK, and one with HSZSN.

TIP FOR SESSIONS WITH OTHERS. Adapt this technique by letting your hands hover over the recipient's crown for a minute or so, and then swipe them down the body slowly. Keep your hands three to four inches away from the body.

Although the chakras can be balanced individually, like everything in the universe, they are interconnected. By bringing balance to one center, you help promote balance in your whole system. A beautiful thing (one of the many) about Reiki is that energy will flow to where it is needed. This also means there is no right or wrong way of doing these practices. The same applies to healing in general. Taking the time to work on your own healing will positively affect everything that surrounds you. In the end, you are the universe and the universe is you.

As for a final tip, just like the Precepts say, during these practices: Do not anger, do not worry, have gratitude, be diligent, be kind to yourself and others, and, last but not least, have fun on this exciting journey! Happy healing!

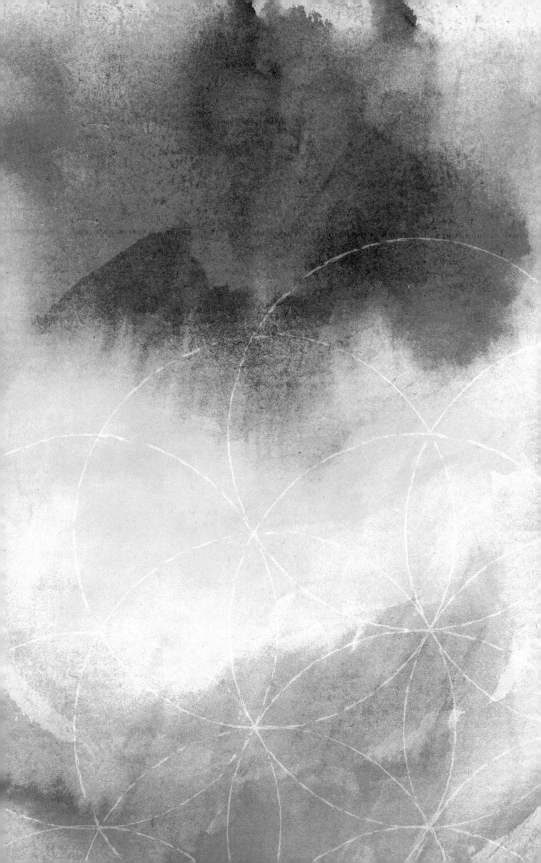

RESOURCES

MUSIC FOR SESSIONS
Deep Relaxation Series by Milkyway Outcast

Hands of Light by Deuter

Liquid Silk by Marina Raye

Soul Sounding byDavid Jesse Kennet

Tao of Healing by Dean Evenson

Tibetan Singing Bowls: Journey into the 7 Chakras by Vidura Barrios, Music for Deep Meditation

BOOKS
Self-Healing with Reiki: How to Create Wholeness, Harmony & Balance for Body, Mind & Spirit by Penelope Quest

The Reiki Sourcebook by Bronwen and Frans Stiene

Wheels of Life by Anodea Judith

REIKI ORGANIZATIONS
Center for Reiki Research

Mid-Atlantic Reiki Conference

Northwest Reiki Gathering

The Reiki Share Project

To search for a Reiki share or circle near you:

Meetup.com

REFERENCES

Eden Energy Medicine. Accessed January 25, 2020. https://www.innersource.net/em/.

Hall, Judy. *Crystals to Empower You.* London: Godsfield Press, 2013.

Jaspar, Nathalie. *Reiki as a Spiritual Practice: An Illustrated Guide.* New York: Dive into Reiki, 2018.

Judith, Anodea. *Eastern Body, Western Mind. Psychology and the Chakra System as a Path to the Self.* New York: Celestial Arts, 2004.

Judith, Anodea. *Wheels of Life: The Classic Guide to the Chakra System (Second Edition).* Minnesota, Woodbury, MN: Llewellyn Publications, 2016.

Heather, Simon. *"Origins of the Chakras." Accessed January 25, 2020. http://www.simonheather.co.uk/ pages/articles/origins_of_the_chakras.pdf.*

Lembo, Margaret Ann. *The Essential Guide to Crystals, Minerals, and Stones.* Woodbury, MN: Llewellyn Publications, 2013.

Quest, Penelope. *Reiki for Life: The Complete Guide to Reiki Practice for Levels 1, 2 & 3.* New York: Tarcher Perigree, 2010.

Quest, Penelope. *Self-Healing with Reiki: How to Create Wholeness, Harmony, and Balance for Body, Mind & Spirit.* London: Penguin Books Ltd., 2003.

Stiene, Bronwen, and Frans Steine. *The Japanese Art of Reiki.* Hants, UK: O Books, 2005.

Stiene, Bronwen and Frans Steine. *The Reiki Sourcebook—Revised and Expanded.* Hants, U.K., 2008.

The Tapping Solution Foundation. Accessed January 25, 2020: https://www.tappingsolutionfoundation.org/.

AILMENTS INDEX

GENERAL INDEX

Heart, 78, 92
Heart chakra, 50–51, 145
  crystals, 111
  emotional, mental, and spiri-
    tual body, 147
  essential oils, 112
  hand positions, 148
  physical body, 146
  symbols and mantras, 149–150
  tapping, 118
  yoga, 120
Heart energy, 34
Heaven energy, 34
Holy Fire Reiki, 12
Hon Sha Ze Sho Nen/HSZSN
    (Distance), 66–67, 70, 114

J

Jikiden Reiki, 12
Joshin Kokyu Ho, 113
Judith, Anodea, 42

K

Karuna Reiki, 10
Kenyoku Ho, 112–113
Ki, 4, 19
Knees, 85, 97
Kundalini, 19–20
Kundalini awakening, 20
Kundalini Reiki, 11

L

Levels, of Reiki, 33–36
Lineage, 20
Lower back, 84, 102

M

Mantras, 20, 70–71
  crown chakra, 171–172
  heart chakra, 149–150
  root chakra, 129–130
  sacral chakra, 136–137
  solar plexus chakra, 143
  third eye chakra, 164–165
  throat chakra, 157–158

Masters, 32–33, 35–37
Meditation, 23, 112–114
Meridians, 21
Middle back, 83, 101
Music, 114–115

N

Navel, 94

P

Past issues, healing, 29
Patanjali, 119
Pets, 106
Plants, 107
Prana, 21

R

Radiant Circuits, 21–22
Rand, William, 10, 12
Reiki
  about, 4–5
  benefits of, 27–29
  elements of, 5
  healing basics, 26–27
  history of, 6–8
  levels of practice, 33–36
  masters, 32–33, 35–37
  Precepts of, 13
  styles of, 9–12
Root chakra, 44–45, 125
  crystals, 111
  emotional, mental, and spiri-
    tual body, 126–127
  essential oils, 111
  hand positions, 127–129
  physical body, 126
  symbols and mantras, 129–130
  tapping, 118
  yoga, 119

S

Sacral chakra, 46–47, 133
  crystals, 111
  emotional, mental, and spiri-
    tual body, 134–135

ACKNOWLEDGMENTS

This book would not have been possible without Crystal Nero and Katie Parr from Callisto Publishing, who put their trust in us. We are so grateful for the awesome opportunity.

I, Nathalie, would love to thank all my teachers, especially Frans Stiene, who pointed the way to a deeper practice and constantly encouraged me to be brutally honest and compassionate at the same time—not always an easy feat. I also count the support of many wonderful family members and friends who have loved me and accepted me no matter what. My Reiki journey would not be the same without you.

I, Alena, would like to thank all of my teachers. I would especially like to acknowledge the sacred cultures of Japan and India for passing down the traditional teachings of Reiki and the chakras, without which our understanding and interpretations would not be possible. I would also like to thank my husband, close family members, and friends, whose support and encouragement have been essential in my healing journey.

ABOUT THE AUTHORS

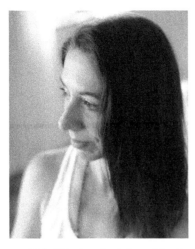

Nathalie Jaspar is a Reiki master with over a decade of experience in the traditional Japanese style. She's a graduate teacher from the International House of Reiki, led by world-renowned Reiki master Frans Stiene. She also trained with the Center for True Health and the International Center for Reiki, and practiced with Reiki master Pamela Miles at the JCC Reiki Clinics in New York. Recently, Nathalie completed a three-week training in Zen meditation and Buddhism at the Chokai-san International Zendo in Akita, Japan.

She is the author of a previous book, *Reiki as a Spiritual Practice: An Illustrated Guide.*

Beyond offering sessions and workshops in NYC, Nathalie has been invited to demo Reiki practice in venues as diverse as Soho House, advertising agencies, Fashion Week events, and the New York Jets' athletic center.

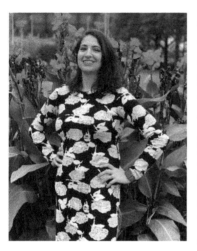 **Alena Goldstein** is a health and wellness professional with a variety of experience in the field. She obtained her master's degree in public health with a specialization in community health education. She has worked for many years researching health promotion and disease prevention, particularly within underserved communities. Over the years, Alena has also dived deeply into holistic and alternative healing. She has trained under Dive Into Reiki and Firefly Society to the level of Reiki Master. In addition, she is a certified integrative nutrition health coach via the Institute for Integrative Nutrition and a 200+ hour yoga instructor via Laughing Lotus, New York City, and more. In 2018, Alena cofounded a not-for-profit initiative, Yoga Share, which seeks to make yoga more inclusive and accessible in NYC. Alena is passionate about holistic healing on all levels—individual, communal, and universal. She offers individual sessions and community classes in New York City.